PROMOTING PARTNERSHIP FOR HEALTH

The Case for Interprofessional Collaboration

In Health and Social Care

Geoffrey Meads
John Ashcroft

with

Hugh Barr
Rosalind Scott
Andrea Wild

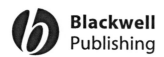

Blackwell
Publishing

CAIPE

© 2005 by Blackwell Publishing Ltd

Editorial offices:
Blackwell Publishing Ltd, 9600 Garsington Road, Oxford OX4 2DQ, UK
    Tel: +44 (0)1865 776868
Blackwell Publishing Inc., 350 Main Street, Malden, MA 02148-5020, USA
    Tel: +1 781 388 8250
Blackwell Publishing Asia Pty Ltd, 550 Swanston Street, Carlton, Victoria 3053, Australia
    Tel: +61 (0)3 8359 1011

First published 2005 by Blackwell Publishing Ltd

Library of Congress Cataloging-in-Publication Data

Meads, Geoff.
  The case for interprofessional collaboration / Geoffrey Meads, John Ashcroft; with Hugh Barr,
Rosalind Scott, Andrea Wild.
       p. ; cm.
  Includes bibliographical references and index.
  ISBN 1-4051-1103-8 (pbk. : alk. paper)
  1. Health care teams. 2. Interprofessional relations. 3. Medical cooperation.
  [DNLM: 1. Patient Care Team. 2. Delivery of Health Care–methods. 3. Interinstitutional Relations.
4. International Cooperation. 5. Interprofessional Relations. W 84.8 M482c 2004] I. Ashcroft, John.
II. Title.

R729.5.H4M43 2004
610.69–dc22   2004009932

ISBN 1-4051-1103-8

A catalogue record for this title is available from the British Library

Set in 10 on 12.5pt Palatino
by Kolam Information Services Pvt. Ltd, Pondicherry, India

The publisher's policy is to use permanent paper from mills that operate a sustainable forestry policy,
and which has been manufactured from pulp processed using acid-free and elementary chlorine-free
practices. Furthermore, the publisher ensures that the text paper and cover board used have met
acceptable environmental accreditation standards.

For further information on Blackwell Publishing, visit our website:
www.blackwellpublishing.com

The opinions expressed in this book are those of the editors and authors concerned. These views are
not necessarily those held by Blackwell Publishing.

Contents

Contributors   iv
The Series   v
Foreword   vii
Preface   ix
Abbreviations   xi
Dedication   xiv

Section one   Policy into Practice
                    Geoffrey Meads and John Ashcroft   1

Chapter one   Introduction   3
Chapter two   Collaboration   15
Chapter three   The Case For   36

Section two   Practice into Policy
                    Rosalind Scott, John Ashcroft and Andrea Wild   59

Chapter four   Crisis Prevention   61
Chapter five   Performance   85
Chapter six   Development   104

Section three   The Professional Experience
                    Geoffrey Meads and Hugh Barr   121

Chapter seven   Personal Learning   123
Chapter eight   Learning Together   135

Section four   Postscript
                    Andrea Wild and Geoffrey Meads   151

Chapter nine   Summing Up   153

Appendices

1 The UK Centre for the Advancement of Interprofessional Education   155
2 The Relationships Foundation   158
3 International Primary Care Unit, University of Warwick   159

Index   161

Contributors

Geoffrey Meads is Professor of Organisational Research in the Division of Health in the Community at the Warwick University Medical School. He chairs the UK Centre for the Advancement of Interprofessional Education and has written widely on developments in health policy and public service relationships.

John Ashcroft is Research Director at the Relationships Foundation in Cambridge, where he leads projects on public service reform and audits of organisational relationships. These have been combined in programmes to evaluate policy implementation and support organisational development in a range of health care organisations.

Hugh Barr is Emeritus Professor of Interprofessional Education in the School of Integrated Health at the University of Westminster, Visiting Professor in Interprofessional Education in the School of Health and Social Care at the University of Greenwich, President of the UK Centre for the Advancement of Interprofessional Education (CAIPE) and Editor-in-Chief of the *Journal of Interprofessional Education*. He was formerly an Assistant Director of the then Central Council for Education and Training in Social Work.

Rosalind Scott currently works for the Law Commission after periods as research assistant at the Movement for Christian Democracy and Relationships Foundation. After graduating in Social and Political Sciences at Cambridge she was a parliamentary secretary and constituency case worker in Bermondsey.

Andrea Wild is a Senior Research Fellow in the Centre for Primary Health Care Studies at the University of Warwick. She has a Social Science degree from Coventry University and a PhD in Social Policy from The University of Warwick.

The Series

Promoting Partnership for Health

Health is everybody's responsibility: individuals, families, communities, professions, businesses, charities and public services. It is more than prevention and cure of disease. It is life-fulfilling for the wellbeing of all. Each party has its role, but effective health improvement calls for partnership, more precisely for many partnerships which bring them together in innovative and imaginative ways. The scope for this series is correspondingly wide.

Successive books will explore partnership for health from policy, practice and educational perspectives. All three drive change. Policy presses the pace of reform everywhere, as this first book in the series demonstrates compellingly. Change is, however, also driven by the demands of practice, triggered by economic and social trends, technological advance and rising public expectations. Education responds but also initiates as a change agent in its own right.

Progressive healthcare is patient centred. The series will wholeheartedly endorse that principle, but the patient is also relative, citizen, client and consumer:

- relative sustaining, and sustained by, family
- citizen working for, and benefiting from, community, country and comity of nations
- client of countless professions
- consumer of health-enhancing or health-harming services

A recurrent theme will be the roles and responsibilities of professions, individually and collectively, to promote and sustain health. The focus will be on the health and social care professions, but taking into account the capability of every profession to improve or impair health. The responsibility of the professions in contemporary society will resonate throughout the series starting from the premise that shared values of professionalism carry an inescapable obligation to further the health and wellbeing of all.

Each book will compare and contrast national perspectives, from developing and so-called developed nations, set within a global appreciation of opportunities and threats to health. Each will be driven, not simply by self-evident scope for one nation to learn from another, but also by the need to respond to challenges that pay no respect to national borders and can only be addressed by concerted action.

Partnership has become so fashionable that it is tempting to assume that all reasonable men and women will unite in common cause. Experience teaches otherwise: best laid plans too often founder for lack of attention to differences which can bedevil relationships between professions and between organisations. This series will not be starry eyed. It will alert readers to the pitfalls and to ways to avoid them.

The three books introducing the series focus on collaborative working and learning between services and between professions in health and social care. The first finds collaboration critical to effective implementation of health care reforms around the world. The second makes the case for interprofessional education as a means to promote collaborative practice corroborated by emerging evidence from systematic searches of the literature. The third marries evidence with experience to assist teachers to develop, deliver and evaluate interprofessional education programmes. All three transcend professional, organisational and national boundaries to share experience as widely as possible for the common good, as they set the tone for the series.

Hugh Barr
Series Editor
Autumn 2004

List of books in the series to follow

Barr, H., Koppel, I., Reeves, S., Freeth, D. & Hammick, M. (Forthcoming) *Effective Inter-professional Education: Argument, Experience and Evidence* ISBN 1 4051 1654 4
Freeth, D., Hammick, M., Barr, H., Koppel, I. & Reeves, S. (Fothcoming) Effective Inter-professioanl Education: Development, Delivery and Evaluation ISBN 1 4051 1653 6

Foreword

Relationships lie at the heart of health and social care. They are a significant factor in our personal health and well-being, while the nature and conduct of a wide range of relationships influences the quality of the care that we receive. However, even with the best intentions it is hard to order our relationships effectively, individually or as a society.

My own interest in how the political, economic and social order shapes relationships goes back to life in Nairobi in the 1970s. Students there were asking whether they should be Marxists, following the violent revolution in neighbouring Ethiopia; or Socialists, following the 'ujamaa' socialism of Julius Nyerere in Tanzania; or follow the more capitalist approach to land reform of Jomo Kenyatta in Kenya. In each country whole systems of relationships were reordered, with very different community outcomes.

This book explores how global modernising policies are reshaping health care relationships. The current UK context is reform, not revolution. Yet health and social care professions are faced with substantial changes in the pattern of their relationships. Both in the UK and internationally, they are part of a political process of seeking wider social and economic outcomes, at the same time as pursuing their own vocation among the individuals, families and communities they serve. Providing health and social care depends upon the quality of professional relationships, and redefines those relationships. In the context of change it is essential to be clear about how to define our goals in terms of relationships, as well as to understanding how we structure and conduct relationships to achieve those goals. For the professions, collaboration in key relationships, and the learning and development which results, is an essential context for this task.

The contribution of the Relationships Foundation to this book is part of a wider programme of work which is seeking to learn how to sustain relationships across society. With respect to public services this has included supporting organisational development in primary care, as well as considering the interplay between public services and changing family and community relationships. Getting the latter right is essential if a focus on relationships is to be the key to tackling the consequences of social alienation.

The message of this book is timely and important. It offers a powerful reminder of the price of failing to get relationships right within our public services. More significantly, it demonstrates the dividends of focusing on relationships, together with lessons and examples of how to achieve these dividends within the current policy context. Thirty years on from those early discussions in Nairobi I still feel, in many ways, a beginner when it comes to the theme of relationships, so I warmly welcome this book as part of a long-term programme of relationships education and management.

Michael Schluter
Chairman, The Relationships Foundation

Preface

Traumatic events do bring people together. Collaboration is often a positive response to adverse circumstances. So it has been with this book. Written by five people with varying levels of past association with the UK Centre for the Advancement of Interprofessional Education (CAIPE), and with each other, the book represents a coming together in response to the terminal illness of the man who should by rights, have been its author.

Paul Gorman died in 2002. Over the three years that he suffered from cancer he continued to plan and hope that he would be able to fulfil his ambition to assist health and social care professionals by providing them with a written guide that would improve the service of their working lives – together. He had already produced a standard text on multidisciplinary teamwork[1]. A passionate believer in collaboration, he would have brought a felicitous style of writing to the subject of interpersonal learning and development, which we cannot emulate, but we have done our best to imitate. This is a book that needs to be readable. Paul's original format for the book, to which we have tried to remain true, was all about offering simple and usable answers to the basic questions posed by those with busy lives in today's ever changing health and social care organisations.

Our purpose is the same. Paul adopted a UK perspective. We go further, recognising that collaboration and its associate issues know no geographical boundaries. This has provided us with the opportunity to draw on current and often previously unpublished research and developments from all over the globe. We hope that this offers a larger tribute to Paul.

There are others, of course, whom we must acknowledge. Those overseas who have arranged and participated in the interviews, site visits, surveys and workshops from which much of our data is derived, are too numerous to mention by name. The same applies back home to those in health and social care organisations we have studied over the past ten years.

But particular thanks are due to our key sponsors and supporters. Amongst the former, Dr John Horder at CAIPE, Dr Michael Schluter at the Relationships Foundation and Dr Frances Griffiths at the Centre for Primary Health Care Studies, University of Warwick, have been pivotal in enlisting their organisations'

---

[1] Originally a historian and urban planner Paul drew together his freelance experience of facilitation with NHS agencies in *Managing Multidisciplinary Teams in the NHS* (1998). Kogan Page, London. His training and consultancy also took him into collaborations with the NSPCC, local authorities, as well as, of course, with CAIPE.

commitment. Amongst the supporters, Dr David Percy at the Special Health Authority, responsible for the NHS university project, Dr Philip Leech and Pippa Bagnall, guardians of interprofessional care at the Department of Health, and Professor Jeremy Dale, at the University of Warwick, have been important personal associates in the UK. Abroad, the quiet facilitative support of UK Embassies, Canning House, the British Council and Department for International Development officers has been too easy to take for granted, with the likes of Michael Valdes Scott, Victoria Harrison, Peter Bird, Ariel Frisancho, Monica Eggers, Paula Santana, Mark Lewis, Alan Richmond, Louise Batchelder, Mamas Tountas, Christos Lionis and Chutatip Siripak not only enabling us to understand globalisation in practice, but to experience its real potential for collaborative goodwill.

Finally, two individuals deserve a special mention for their behind the scenes spadework: Michiyo Iwami and Catherine Beckett. Their research and adminis-tration has contributed to every page of the text, and we are deeply grateful.

Collaborative enterprise is hard work, often without tangible reward or visible result. We hope all who have helped us will feel, along with Paul Gorman's family, that this book does offer such an outcome.

Geoffrey Meads
Highcroft, Winchester
Autumn 2004

Abbreviations

AANP	American Academy of Nurse Practitioners
AIDS	Acquired Immune Deficiency Syndrome
ANZAME	Australia and New Zealand Association for Medical Education
APMCG	National Association of General Medical Practitioners (Portugal)
BLAT	British Life Assurance Trust
BMJ	British Medical Journal
BRHSC	Bristol Royal Hospital for Sick Children
CAIPE	Centre for the Advancement of Interprofessional Education
CBHD	Community-Based Health Development (Philippines)
CHAI	Commission for Health Audit and Inspection
CHD	Coronary Heart Disease
CHI	Commission for Health Improvement
CHW	Community Health Worker
CLAS	Comités Locales de Administración de Salud (Peru)
COBES	Community-Based Education and Service
COME	Community Oriented Medical Education
CRIS	Crime Information System
CVD	Cardiovascular Disease
DETR	Department of Environment, Transport and the Regions
DFID	Department for International Development
DOH	Department of Health
DRG	Diagnostic Related Group
DTC	Diagnostic and Treatment Centre
EMPE	European Network for the Development of Multi-Professional Education in Health Sciences
EPS	Entidades Promotoras de Salud (Colombia)
ESS	Empresas Solidarias de Salud (Colombia)
EU	European Union
EYS	National Health System (Greece)
FONASA	Health Fund (Chile)
GDP	Gross Domestic Product
GITT	Geriatric Interdisciplinary Team Training
GP	General Practitioner
GPWSI	General Practitioner With Special Interest
HAZ	Health Action Zone
HEA	Health Education Authority

HIV	Human Immunodeficiency Virus
HMO	Health Maintenance Organisation
HPSISNP	Health Professions Schools in Service to the Nation Program
HSC	Health Service Circular
IKA	Ministry of Social Affairs (Greece)
IMSS	National Insurance Fund (Mexico)
IPE	Interprofessional Education
IPPR	Institute of Public Policy Research
ISAPRE	Private Insurance Fund (Chile)
IT	Information Technology
JET	Joint Evaluation Team
KELA	National Social Security Institute (Finland)
LHB	Local Health Board (Philippines)
LHS	Local Health System
LSP	Local Strategic Partnership
MINSA	Ministry of Health (Peru)
NGO	Non-Governmental Organisation
NHS	National Health Service (UK)
NHSU	National Health Service University
NICE	National Institute for Clinical Excellence
NIPNET	Nordic Interprofessional Network
NIVEL	Netherlands Institute of Primary Health Care
NSF	National Service Framework
OECD	Organisation for Economic Cooperation and Development
PAHO	Pan-American Health Organisation
PALS	Patient Advocacy and Liaison Services
PBL	Problem/Patient-Based Learning
PCG	Primary Care Group
PCS	Paediatric Cardiac Surgery
PCT	Primary Care Trust
PEST	Political, Economic, Social, Technological
POS	Compulsory Insurance Plan (Colombia)
PIU	Performance and Innovation Unit
PMS	Primary Medical Services
RCGP	Royal College of General Practitioners
RSM	Royal Society of Medicine
SARS	Severe Acute Respiratory Syndrome
SRSAG	Supra-Regional Service Advisory Group
SSD	Social Services Department
STAKES	National Institute of Research and Development (Finland)
SUS	Unified Health System (Brazil)
SWAP	Sector-Wide Approach
TUFH	Towards Unity For Health
UBHT	United Bristol Hospitals Trust
UK	United Kingdom

UNESCO	United Nations Educational, Scientific and Cultural Organisation
UNICEF	United Nations Children's Fund
UNI-SOL	Universities in Solidarity for the Health of the Disadvantaged
USA	United States of America
USAID	United States of America International Aid
WFME	World Federation of Medical Education
WHO	World Health Organization
WONCA	World Organisation of National Colleges and Academies (of General Practice)

PAUL GORMAN
In memoriam

Section I
Policy into Practice

In this section we identify the ideas which are influential in shaping collaborative health and social care approaches internationally, and examine models for interprofessional learning and development in the UK.

Geoffrey Meads and John Ashcroft

1 Introduction

Beginnings

This is a book for self-conscious beginners. It is principally for those in the early stages of their careers as health and social care professionals learning to collaborate. It is also for managers and teachers, to guide them in commissioning and providing programmes to promote collaboration.

Being a professional today means becoming interprofessional. It is a policy imperative, demanding behavioural change and sometimes transformation.

This is our starting point: a comprehensive range of new professional career paths matched by modernising strategies for more collaborative relationships. Clinical governance, public health improvement programmes, integrated and intermediate care regimes are all illustrations of such strategies. Each of these is now the subject of articulate and well argued central policies in many countries. But policies alone cannot ensure behavioural change, which begins not so much with collective target groups and government performance priorities as with positive personal understanding, motivation and commitment. Strategies can explain how to progress. They may answer questions about whom, when and where, but they do not, by definition, address questions about why and what for? These are the first order questions, which this book endeavours to answer as it makes the case for collaboration.

Converting collaborative policies into action should begin, for each professional, by re-examining personal principle and self interest. It has to be the right thing to do and it has to be done correctly. This is still the essence of what it means to be a professional: being both ethical and expert[1]. Collaboration starts from these two criteria and works to strengthen both. Interprofessional learning and development needs to add value, in both the moral and economic senses of the term.

Accordingly, this book is designed to serve as a primer on policies which depend upon collaboration for their effective delivery in practice. It begins with the assumption that such collaboration knows no boundaries. Its perspectives and data sources are deliberately international, recognising that with globalisation all

---

[1] Indeed many students of professions argue that the increased complexity of technocratic health care combined with resource constraints and consumer-style demand mean that health and social care professionals must demonstrate they are actually becoming more expert and more ethical to retain public credibility and confidence. See e.g. Southon and Braithwaite (1998) and Harrison (1999).

types of modern health systems now place a premium on closer working relationships between professionals (and non-professionals, as well). Many of the best examples of policies for partnership today come from the economically underdeveloped and developing countries, from which the so-called developed countries such as the UK and the USA have much to learn. As we have described elsewhere[2], in such countries as the Philippines, Mexico and Greece, modernising policies mean that virtually all public service health professionals have to collaborate with representatives from other care professions in municipalities, nongovernmental organisations, private clinics, mixed status foundation hospitals and a multitude of local community projects and cooperative ventures, during the course of a typical working month.

These health professionals increasingly find themselves employed across a spectrum of such settings, as the range of health care contracting agencies expands. Universal modernising policies for multiple funding and stakeholder health care enterprises are inextricably tied to developments in interprofessional collaboration. They are mutually dependent: the motivation to collaborate comes from appreciating what modernisation really means. Accordingly, this is a term to which we return regularly in the pages which follow.

This book also represents a fresh beginning in its choice of evidence from which to examine interprofessional collaboration. It does not confine itself to a rehearsal of recent formal policies for human resources development, important though some of these undoubtedly are.

In the UK, for example, the following assertion by national Government was a watershed statement of authentically new, twenty-first century, epoch-making proportions.

> 'It (modernisation) is about looking at the workforce in a different way, as teams of people rather than as different professional tribes. For too long we have planned and trained staff in a uni-professional/uni-disciplinary way without a clear and comprehensive look at the future.'
>
> (Hargadon & Staniforth, 2000, 1.3)

Declarations such as this are important ingredients of behavioural change, especially in relation to structural developments. The UK Government statement led directly to the establishment of a national network of Workforce Development Confederations to integrate budgetary and planning systems for all (non-medical) health professionals' training; and indirectly to the rapid growth of interprofessional postgraduate curricula in British universities. But policy declarations only tell part of the story. They are not proof of behavioural change and, while easily accessible and superficially attractive, they cannot of themselves supply a convincing case for interprofessional collaboration.

---

[2] This chapter and several subsequent sections of the book draw on fieldwork undertaken by the International Primary Care Unit at the University of Warwick. This work has been described in a series of eight articles for *Primary Care Report* (Medicom Publishers) between December 2002 and July 2004.

In the past, this has customarily meant little more than teamwork. Indispensable though teamwork remains, it is an insufficient basis on which to build contemporary models for collaboration. While the literature on collaboration now extends well beyond teamwork as it embraces the modernisation agenda, evaluations of other models for collaboration remain few and systematic reviews are conspicuous by their absence.

The lack of systematic evaluations of collaboration weakens the evidence base for interprofessional education. More progress has been made in securing the evidence base for interprofessional education, calling on the methodology devised and tested by the Interprofessional Education Joint Evaluation Team (JET) as reported by Barr *et al.* in a later volume in this series.

Whilst recognising the importance of earlier sources, this book locates interprofessional learning and development firmly within its contemporary policy framework. Our primary sources are drawn from the modernisation of health and social care systems, including numerous examples too recent to have reported findings for systematic evaluation, if and when built in.

Our time period for data collection is the decade beginning in 1993, when the World Bank's Development Report recognised that modernising health systems was as critical to long-term economic growth and development as it is to successful social policies[3]. For this period our principal sources of data are the evidence and experience we have accumulated ourselves on interprofessional collaboration through our involvement as facilitators, fieldworkers, consultants and observers in the processes of health systems modernisation. These sources are listed in Table 1.1, with the concluding Appendices providing details of our host organisations and some of their recent activities and publications.

While the footnotes and bibliographies of textual references that close each chapter, and recommendations for further reading together represent a comprehensive guide to the existing theory and practice of interprofessional collaboration, the chapters themselves focus on the preconditions that now prevail for this collaboration in contemporary patterns of organisational and cultural change. The principal evidence includes the findings of new and previously unreported recent collaborative programmes listed in Table 1.1. These encompass case studies of new primary care organisations and their policies across 12 countries; long-term domestic development and international mediation projects involving professional and public service leaderships in such countries as South Africa, Scotland and Rwanda; recent reviews of relevant national inquiries and regulatory reports and most important, the lessons learnt by CAIPE itself, which has been the principal pioneer for innovation and quality in interprofessional collaboration in the UK, and often beyond, during the ten years under review.

These, then, are our beginnings. To summarise: we are writing for new health and social care professionals, their managers and teachers. We are writing about new mindsets and the behavioural changes they can bring. To do this we are

---

[3] *Investing in Health* was a true watershed document. The World Bank is by some way the largest external donor and prior to 1993 its overwhelming focus had been on support just for wealth producing market mechanisms in the commercial and manufacturing sectors (World Bank, 1993).

Table 1.1 Original sources.

Programme	Sponsor	Research Data
International Primary Care	Health Foundation PPP Medical Trust UK Department of Health NHS West Midlands Research Network	transferable learning from 12 global case studies and fieldwork interviews covering: – health and social care combinations – local engagement models – community health partnerships – interprofessional collaboration
International Mediation and Relational Health Care	Relationships Foundation Concordis International	• crisis resolution in political and civil society breakdowns in Africa • relationship audits and development programmes for new NHS partnerships • review of national health care inquiries and regulatory developments, 1972–2002
Interprofessional Learning and Development Programmes (UK)	Centre for the Advancement of Interprofessional Education	• questionnaire survey of recent local quality assurance initiatives in UK • literature review • action research and local projects

utilising new material and new frameworks for promoting interprofessional collaboration. These are rooted in the political concept of modernisation and its practical expressions. It is to this concept that we turn our attention in the remaining sections of this chapter.

Subsequent chapters

The following chapters have a consistent format. Each has an introductory preamble and statement of purpose, balanced by a closing assessment and analysis of the implications for the future design and evaluation of interprofessional learning and development programmes, with a set of conclusions. In between, the principal matter for consideration by readers forms the body of the chapter.

Each chapter utilises the following framework for professional relationships:

- With same profession
- With other professions

- With (new) partners
- With policy actors (in many different guises)
- With public (representatives)
- With patients (and their proxies)

It is a simple list, but it is also very much one that belongs to the new professionalism.

Collaboration is not new. It has always been practised more or less effectively as it is today. It has, however, become more complex and more difficult over the years. Personal and public trust is harder to earn in the context of larger and more competitive organisations with more effective bureaucratic controls.

Risk assessment, performance management and (evidence-based) quality improvement are now the three pillars of (inter) professional accountability. Collaboration is the fundamental requirement within each and across them all. Accordingly the three chapters of Section two of this book examine these three drivers for behavioural change. They adopt an essentially functional paradigm: to seek collaborative advantage is to acknowledge that collaboration for many health professionals is the bottom line of their practice. The raw material of these chapters reflects this perspective: national inquiries, mandatory monitoring requirements and the development agendas arising from (often excessive) clinical and care demand management.

Section two refers back to the remaining two chapters in Section one. In the first of these, a series of analytical models are offered, providing an up-to-date account of collaboration theory. In the next, this is expanded and examined through examples of global developments. The thread that pulls these chapters and the two sections of the book together is functionality. Everything relates back to the specialist skills and tasks of each health and social care profession, which this book seeks to enhance.

In Section three, chapters seven and eight bring together the learning at two levels. Chapter seven concentrates on the lessons for individual professionals and professions. Chapter eight links mounting concern to improve collaboration to the promotion and development of interprofessional education worldwide, as a prelude to the next two books in the series.

These perspectives go hand in hand. Interprofessional collaboration and its particular requirements and forms are, above all, contextual. They can only be understood in their own settings. Chapter nine closes the book with a short summary of the case for collaboration across these settings and points the way for those interested to further enquiry.

Modernisation

At the heart of modernisation is cultural change. This arises from a new political paradigm in which health and health care is recognised as a universal human right and these fundamental responsibilities lie with government (at different levels in different places). The profound intention of the cultural change is to instil collaboration as normative to professional conduct, across the entire new patterns of professional relationships. Modernisation itself is understood in the programmes from which we are drawing our principal data to incorporate five thematics of health systems development. These are as follows:

- local resource management (or decentralisation)
- governance (with new forms of independent regulation)
- integration (based on cross boundary partnerships)
- stewardship for public health (and thence community development)
- quality (linking evidence-based health care to choice and consumerism)

The above apply as much to market oriented health systems as they do to, for example, those which are neo-socialist developments. For all health professionals they are today's facts of life[4].

Of course, each thematic or principle is expressed differently in different places. Local resource management, for example, is invariably about strengthening the legitimacy of decision-making processes regarding intervention options and priorities, especially where resources are scarce. Decentralisation often brings the added benefits for health professionals of additional resources to call on in balancing the decision-making equation. In the Philippines, for example, over the past ten years, the municipal contribution to health care expenditure has risen to virtually the same level as that of the national government (20% in 2002–2003), with consequent benefits in terms of access to lying-in beds, vaccines and volunteer sanitarians. But, there is a downside. Filipino health professionals now have to make decisions knowing that co-paying local mayors and their electors often have views of their own, for example, on family planning and mental health therapies. This can be uncomfortable. The political view, on abortion, for example, may even be perceived as a direct threat to clinical autonomy and patient privacy. The dilemmas that arise, as a result, require new levels of collaborative relationships to ensure that decisions are still made with the degrees of explanation and openness that can sustain professional ethics.

Decentralisation of decision making may be to municipalities as in the Philippines, or even more explicitly in Finland and Sweden where local taxation contributes over 80% of public health expenditure. It may be at regional or provincial levels when part of a long-standing federal system, as in Germany, Canada or Australia. In these countries responsibility for health is understood through 'bottom-up' perspectives which are taken further in such states as Bolivia, Switzerland and Peru where, increasingly, it is community organisations themselves

---

[4] For those wishing to explore the theoretical analyses and political commentaries that have come together in the making of the Modernisation movement, the writings of Peter Drucker, Robert Putnam, Will Hutton and Anthony Giddens provide an excellent introduction and insights. Key references are provided in the chapter's bibliography.

that control the health system as part of wider 'civil society' movements. In Peru, for example, the 1200 Comités Locales Administraciónes de Salud (CLAS) are account-able for over a quarter of the country's health care expenditure. Rooted in local women's and indigenous people's movements in each, there is a locally elected seven-person community management group headed by the lead local health professional. Its powers extend to deciding local prescription charges, vitamin suppliers and clinic sites. For the doctor or nurse-in-charge collaboration is now the modus operandi with vertical line management a memory from past days of dictatorship.

Local resource management can also be implemented through decentralised paying agencies as with the insurance funds in the Netherlands, Israel and Greece or, as in New Zealand, the UK and Thailand, it may be through provider primary care organisations. In the NHS primary care trusts of England a legal 'duty of partnership' now applies and general practitioners are compelled to collaborate in a range of statutory committees with social workers, nurses, other family health service professionals and both patient and elected public representatives[5]. Corpo-racy is obligatory.

Combining individual clinical accountability with collective responsibilities is now the collaborative challenge of governance for health professionals. Govern-ance implies a new parity between professionals, as all are accountable not only for their personal duties but also for the performance of the overall programmes of which they are part. Improvements in the former must contribute to the latter. The behavioural changes required are considerable, from better emphasis on teamwork to new arrangements for 'whistle-blowing', as we shall see in Chapter four.

Governance is a concept that recognises the growing range of legitimate inter-ests in health care. Their effective integration as stakeholders through, for example, collaborative network or learning organisational models can and should mean more effective integration of service delivery and the patient or client experience. Modernisation means that such integration is no longer constrained by boundaries between, in particular, individual professions. Care management, shared protocols, individual need assessments, managed care, intermediate care and care pathways are all new practice concepts of essentially interprofessional collaboration. Each has its stakeholder sponsors: from patient pressure groups for care management to life science companies and independent research institutes for managed care and care pathways. Integration and governance go together and are critical constituents in the case for collaboration.

So too, finally, are the last two thematics of modernising health systems: public health and quality improvement. In both cases the key collaborative relationships for progress are those of professionals in different sectors with each other but, more important, with non-professionals. In such countries as Kenya and Georgia the direction of health care is decided in both a daily operational sense, as well as strategically, by the effectiveness of collaborative arrangements with individual

---

[5] This was prefaced by the New Labour Government's first major NHS policy statement after it came to power in 1997 (Secretary of State, 1997), and subsequently enacted in legislation in the 1999 Health Act.

non-governmental organisations (NGOs) and their regional and national coordinating panels. In 2002 it was their sponsorship in Nairobi which allowed the establishment of a national organisation for general practice, while in Tbilisi it is combined World Bank and European Union tenders which are similarly, in 2004, looking to offer the opportunity for curricula development in gatekeeping family medicine. In other countries the NGO sector is less significant than such other public services as education or transport, while virtually everywhere, and especially in post-Soviet states, the private sector is becoming a more valued collaborator. The model for the latter is, of course, North America where, for example, in the USA alone health professionals have had to relate to more than 50 separate agencies on new health technology assessments[6], and about the same number of new health maintenance organisations. In Portugal the quasi-independent Institute for Quality in Health-Care at Coimbra comprises rotating seconded lead health professionals alongside counterparts from the academic, commercial and political sectors; while its post-1995 14 national health improvement programmes actually derive from combined Interior and Finance Ministry policies designed to integrate the take up of preventive health care and screening with new job training and welfare benefit programmes. In the UK health professionals have responded quickly to the political challenges posed by the new policy emphases on quality and health that possess the intrinsic capacity to empower, for example, businesses, consumer and disadvantaged groups and scientific institutes. Sensing that the dominance of individual professions' national representative bodies is no longer secure, especially in primary care, they have entered into new cross-profession political pacts such as the NHS Alliance and National Association for Primary Care, often culling monetary support from independent sector collaborators (e.g. Medicom, Health and Nuffield Foundations, Pfizer and Glaxo-Wellcome) keen to be associated positively with the new 'duty of partnership'[7].

The five thematics of modernisation can be understood as all powerful determinants of a new collaborative culture for health professionals – across the full and expanding range of their interprofessional functions. The next chapter examines these, but before moving on let us close this chapter by briefly revisiting what modernisation means for the sixfold framework of professional relationships that we described earlier as the backbone for this book.

(1) **With own profession**
    More differentiated roles and terms of employment; practice rather than practitioner contracts; peer review mechanisms and population plus personal list responsibilities; probity and private sector alternatives

(2) **With other professions**
    Shared referrals and procedures; larger multi-specialist service delivery teams; substitution and new skill mix; joint service management; professional

---

[6] This was fifty-three at one count in 1995 and still growing (Perry & Thamer, 1997).

[7] This has now been embedded in two pieces of legislation, the 1999 *Health Act* and the 2002 *NHS Reform and Health Care Professions Act*.

standards regulation and combined development strategies; integrated curricula; and clinical audits

(3) **With new partners**
Sponsorship and shared data systems; joint investments and risk taking;
external consultancy and education; hybrid organisational shapes and status;
new service terms and titles; mixed income streams and multiple accountabilities, including voluntary, private and commercial agencies

(4) **With policy actors**
Innovation and increasing pilot/pioneer programmes; participative forums;
knowledge management; links to devolved political units and pressure
groups; advocacy and (government) agent roles; decision making on health
care options and priorities

(5) **With public**
Extended and more specialist mechanisms of representation and media,
forums of civil society and participatory democracy; community-campus
partnerships; publicly available performance comparators; community
health and social capital gains; NGOs and locally elected representatives
with (health) related roles; independent regulators of the public interest
and auditors

(6) **With patients**
Informed consumers and citizenship movements; litigation and wider direct
access, negotiation and doing deals; contributory and co-payment systems;
combined initiatives and community leadership opportunities; team-based
care and new covenants; incorporation of social care into holistic concept of
health; plus advocates and care managers for patients and carers.

It is clear, from this inventory, that separation is no longer viable for health
professionals. Separation was bound to a sense of independence which, at its
best, has been a reflection of the integrity to which all health professionals
should aspire and, at its worst, is still a symptom of self-seeking status. Collaboration is now the way forward and both integrity and status will be with
those health and social care professionals who independently decide to take this
route.

Lessons

Chapter six explores in detail the transferable learning from course and curricula
innovations arising from the development agendas across international health
systems. At this stage, therefore, we will limit ourselves to just three lessons as a
means of highlighting how the dynamic of modernisation, which we have considered in this opening chapter, is creating the preconditions for collaborative

behavioural change through new interprofessional learning and development. Deliberately, these are selected from very different cultural settings.

First, in northern Kenya at the University of Eldoret, the home town of past President Moi, there is the Community-Based Education and Service Programme (COBES). All trainee doctors and nurses are required to spend at least three weeks per annum located at a community health facility. This is as part of a continuous programme of placements allowing the university and local population to be in a continuous relationship. As a result students do not simply have the chance to test and extend their skills outside hospital but also to be integral to the process of identifying and responding to local needs. These have ranged from malaria netting and HIV education to new water jars, latrines and granaries. The COBES collaboration is now regarded rightly as an 'anchor organisation' of the Kenyan health system.

At Chisinău in Moldova the Medical School is engaged in a major Primary Health Care Education programme designed to underpin a fundamental restructuring of the previous multi-specialist, Shemasko polyclinic system. The twin targets are the conversion to family practice of internists, paediatricians, physicians and a number of other previously hospital-based doctors, and the establishment of community nursing – all within an overall framework of interprofessional learning. The latter has been supplied by the University of Helsinki. The specifications for the curricula change came from Spain and England as part of a European Union sponsored consultancy. NGO sponsorship has been USA based through Carelift International and the participating Moldovan health professionals have been linked to counterparts undergoing a similar process at Vilnius and Kaunas Universities in Lithuania. Modernisation in Moldova is a classic contemporary collaboration.

In the UK in 2002 the Government supplied a considerable boost to interprofessional collaboration through a grant of £25 million for the development of university curricula in the following three new subject areas, under the banner of 'modernising education':

- Common learning programmes for all health professionals in communications and NHS principles
- Changing workforce practices and effective ways of working together
- Integration across professional and organisational boundaries (and barriers)

Four pilot sites were selected for special funding, each comprising two or more universities in partnership with neighbouring health and social care agencies and supported by Workforce Development Confederations. They were Southampton and Portsmouth universities, Newcastle, Northumbria and Sunderland universities, Sheffield and Sheffield Hallam universities, and King's College London, with Greenwich and London South Bank universities. These are just some of the many 'pre-registration common learning sites' established nationwide, funded through Workforce Development Confederations.

Problem-Based Learning (PBL) is one of many methods introduced into such programmes, advocated, amongst others, by the University of Limburg at Maastricht in the Netherlands where, amongst many interprofessional education programmes, nine local community committees work with individual cardiologist and general practitioner pairings to identify, negotiate access to and treat (up to 3000) targeted individuals at risk of coronary heart disease. Such initiatives encapsulate the new pattern of relationships required of health professionals, embracing collaboration right across the six headings of our standard framework[8].

Conclusions

This chapter has both introduced the structure of this book and illustrated its processes. The two are interrelated but interdependent. Collaboration is delivered through interprofessional learning and development. Modernising policies entail new approaches to that collaboration. The chapter, in its evidence and sources, international perspectives and focus on the organisational and cultural preconditions for behavioural change and transformation, has sought to epitomise one such approach.

Bibliography

Barr, H., Koppel, I., Reeves, S., Freeth, D. & Hammick, M. (Forthcoming) *Effective Interprofessional Education: Argument, Assumption and Evidence*. Blackwell, Oxford.

Drucker, P. (1994) *Post-Capitalist Society*. Butterworth-Heinemann, Oxford.

Giddens, A. (1998) *The Third Way. The Renewal of Social Democracy*. Polity Press, London.

Hargadon, J. & Staniforth, M. (2000) *A Health Service of all the Talents: Developing the NHS Workforce*. Department of Health, London.

Hutton, W. (2000) *New Life for Health*. The Commission on the NHS (Chair). Vintage, London.

Meads, G., Iwami, M. & Wild, A. (2002–2004) International Primary Care Series. *Primary Care Report*, Medicom, London.

Perry, S. & Thamer, M. (1997) Health technology assessment: Decentralised and fragmented in the United States compared to other countries. *Health Policy*, **40**, 177–98.

Putnam, R. D. (1993) *Making Democracy Work: Civic Tradition in Modern Italy*. Princeton University Press, New Jersey.

Secretary of State for Health (1999) *Health Act*. The Stationery Office, London.

Secretary of State for Health (2002) *NHS Reform and Health Care Professions Act*. The Stationery Office, London.

---

[8] The Bibliography contains source references for each of the new educational initiatives and ideas cited in this chapter, plus further examples that readers may wish to explore.

Further Reading

Barr, H. (2002) *Interprofessional Education. Today, Yesterday and Tomorrow*. Learning and Teaching Support Network for Health Sciences and Practice, Occasional Paper No. 1. King's College London.

Bivol, G., Curichin, G., Sutnick, A. *et al.* (2002) Development of Family Medicine Education in Moldova with Carelift International. *Education for Health*, **15** (2), 202–14.

Freeth, D., Hammick, M., Barr, H. Koppel, I. & Reeves, S. (Forthcoming) *Effective Interprofessional Education: Development, Delivery and Evaluation*. Blackwell, Oxford.

Freeth, D., Hammick, M., Koppel, I., Reeves, S. & Barr, H. (2002) *A Critical Review of Evaluations of Interprofessional Education*. Learning and Teaching Support Network for Health Sciences and Practice, Occasional Paper No. 2, King's College London.

Harrison, S. (1999) Clinical autonomy and health policy: past and futures. In: *Professionals and the New Managerialism* (eds M. Exworthy & S. Halford), pp. 50–56. Open University Press, Buckingham.

Secretary of State for Health (1997) *The New NHS. Modern, Dependable*. The Stationery Office, Cm 3807, London.

Southon, G. & Braithwaite, J. (1998) The end of professionalism? *Social Science and Medicine*, **46** (1), 23–8.

World Bank (1993) *Investing in Health*. World Bank, Geneva.

Zwarenstein, M., Atkins J., Barr H., Hammick M., Koppelm I. & Reeves, S. (1999) A systematic review of interprofessional education. *Journal of Interprofessional Care*, **13**, 4, 417–24.

2 Collaboration

Terms of reference

What is collaboration? Many countries are reforming and modernising their health and social care services, seeking to instil the culture of collaboration within appropriate structures and processes. The previous chapter has described how five themes of health service development – local resource management, governance, integration, stewardship for public health, and quality – together represent a political, organisational and educational imperative for collaboration. This chapter seeks to give some more detailed substance to the term 'collaboration', describing and defining what it is. The chapter recognises the reality of both the obstacles as well as the dividends that can accrue from effective collaboration.

The language of relationships can be slippery and nebulous. Warm fuzzy words can mask a complex and, at times, painful reality. This chapter draws specifically on work of the Relationships Foundation[1], a Cambridge based 'think and do tank', in reviewing and supporting the development of organisational relationships in many sectors. We will start by considering four key questions before examining their implications for the key collaborative relationships that structure much of the content of this book:

- What is collaboration?
- How can collaborative relationships be analysed?
- What are the dividends of collaboration?
- How can collaboration deal with difference?

What is collaboration?

At its simplest collaboration is about working together. It therefore implies both difference (it is something less than complete integration or unification), and commonality (there is some shared goal or activity which is the focus of collaboration). Collaboration is also about relationships – working together and not just alongside. It implies more than activities which overlap or interact in some way

---

[1] www.relationshipsfoundation.org Details of the role of the Foundation are contained in Appendix 2 at the end of this book.

and would normally include some conscious interaction between the parties to achieve a common goal. However, an individual's actions may be interpreted by others as part of a broader collaborative endeavour whether or not the individual sees his or her contribution in this light.

In setting out the case for collaboration it will be helpful to begin by exploring something of the range of meaning that collaboration can convey, and some of the key concepts associated with the term. A number of aspects of collaboration and examples of their expression are summarised in Table 2.1. In seeking to unpack the concept of collaboration it is helpful for professionals to distinguish the functional and transformative purposes of collaboration[2]. Much of this book depicts collaboration as a rational strategy to achieve certain goals. The possible rationales for collaboration are explored in more detail later in the chapter. It is, however, important to note that the process of collaboration may change (intentionally or otherwise) the participants, empowering individuals and communities and strengthening civil society[3]. We also explore these developmental goals, noting that internationally these may be an important policy objective in themselves.

The specific goals of collaboration vary according to the level at which collaboration takes place. This has recently been explored with respect to emerging public health networks in London, where different relational interactions at strategic, executive, operational and technical levels could be distinguished (Shaw *et al.*, 2002). Collaboration is needed to ensure strategic coherence of goals and priorities. Such coherence requires collaboration between executives of relevant agencies to create the organisational context for operational collaboration in the delivery of services. This needs to be complemented by technical collaboration (in this case within public health networks), where technical expertise distributed amongst a range of professions and organisations can be brought together for the

Table 2.1 A taxonomy of collaboration.

Aspects of collaboration	Examples of their expression
Goal	Functional or transformational
Level	Strategic, executive, operational, technical
Process	Cooperation, coordination, exchange, sharing
Structure	Networks, teams, pathways, partnerships, area based initiatives, merged organisations
Power and influence	Participation, empowerment, co-option and control, infiltration and subversion
Proximity	In time and/or space
Duration	Temporary task focused or longer term strategy
Complexity	Bipolar or multipolar

---

[2] A helpful discussion of both of these aspects can be found in Huxham (1996).

[3] See, for example, Estlund (2003) on the potential of workplace bonds to strengthen civil society or Wilkinson & Appelbee (1999) and Nash (2002) on strengthening community. See also Chapter three, pp. 52–54.

benefit of a number of organisations. An individual may be involved in relationships at more than one level.

The various goals of collaboration can be expressed in different processes
surrounding the flow and utilisation of, for example, finance, time, skills or
information. These processes may be formal organisational processes and
working practices, or the product of more informal interpersonal interactions.
The range of processes is also indicated in the variety of ways in which a
particular goal can be described. So, for example, the goal of greater continuity
of care can be discussed in terms of the continuum of care (in disease management), coordination of care, discharge planning, case management, integration of
services and seamless care (Haggerty *et al.*, 2003). Some would want to reserve the
term 'collaboration' for a closer degree of mutual involvement and so distinguish
it from lower level interactions such as coordinating activity. Others are willing to
use the term more broadly, recognising that there may be different levels of
commitment and degrees of involvement in different collaborative relationships.
Our interest here is not so much in the semantics of the term 'collaboration' but to
note that different transactional processes will be appropriate or sufficient in
different contexts. These may reflect the levels of ambition of the agreed goals.

These processes may be expressed in different structures, and indeed the
creation of new structures may be one of the outcomes of collaboration which
reflects the maturation and deepening of the relationship (or the requirements of
policy). Networks and teams tend to be more focused on the interpersonal aspects
of collaboration, though crossing disciplinary and organisational boundaries, and
typically focused around a task, goal or function. Partnerships are often focused
on single issues or client groups (for example smoking cessation, teenage pregnancy, drugs, mental health) but assume greater organisational form with dele-
gated budgets and responsibilities. Area based initiatives have a geographic
rather than issue/client-group focus[4], although they retain many of the characteristics of partnerships. The emergence of joint service providers in the form of
combined health and social care trusts in the UK illustrates the potential for
collaborative working arrangements to be adopted in new organisational forms.

Collaboration involves different degrees of power and influence and can be
seen as alternative ways of responding to those differences. In looking at
new organisational developments in primary care in the UK we found few people
who felt that they held the power in their health care relationships[5]. This was in
part a consequence of such different types of power as financial control, regulatory or sapiential authority, political influence, local legitimacy and control of
delivery.

Those who controlled the budgets did not necessarily control delivery of
services and were held accountable for the performance of others over whom

---

[4] The selection of the geographic area may, or course, be influenced by the concentration of particular
needs in that area.

[5] See our earlier volume based on emerging interprofessionally-led NHS primary care groups, Meads
& Ashcroft (2000).

they felt they had, at times, limited influence (the UK 'market' at the time being characterised by very limited provider plurality). Informal network influence may be more powerful than the formally designated lines of control and accountability. In the context of differences in power, collaboration can be used positively to encourage and empower participation. But collaboration can become the forum for power games – being used to co-opt and control potentially destabilising forces, or be seen as a strategy for subverting other people's agendas.

Collaboration can involve different degrees of proximity in time or space. It may be sequential, with the focus on joining the different steps to provide a package of seamless care. So, for example, an acute (hospital) trust and social services department may collaborate around the discharge of an elderly patient with little overlap of their caregiving functions. Collaboration can also be co-located and concurrent with people physically working together on the same overall task at more or less the same time. A nurse and doctor may, for example, work together at the same bedside. Collaboration can also be found in virtual relationships, perhaps most often in the context of research and learning, where the focus is on the exchange of ideas and information, where activities conducted at the same time but in different places can be brought together for added benefit.

Collaboration also varies in its duration and complexity. At its simplest it involves two parties in a bipolar relationship. However, even if a bipolar relationship can be identified, it will normally be part of a wider system with the bipolar collaborative relationships being influenced by what happens in the other relationships to which one or other is party. At its most complex these other relationships are drawn into a multi-party collaborative endeavour. Collaboration can represent a long-term strategic commitment but may also apply to time-limited task-focused joint work. A specific example of collaboration may be short-lived, but part of a much wider and longer-term collaborative process. Thus the nature of collaboration can be very different according to the context.

Analysing collaboration

Health and social care involves many different relationships. This variety of relationships, developed in very different contexts, makes analysis of collaborative relationships difficult. The variety of forms of collaboration compounds the difficulty. In helping health care and other organisations to think through their collaborative relationships we have found it helpful in our research and development work to ask the following questions:

(1) **Who do I need to work with now and in the future?**
     Sometimes participation in a relationship is determined by the task and context. There may be a choice as to whether or not the relationship is regarded as collaborative, but working together in some way is necessary and unavoidable. At other times the choice of possible collaborative relationships

far exceeds the number of relationships that can be effectively developed and maintained. In working with new primary care organisations in the UK to assess their strategic relationships in promoting public health many groups struggled to keep their list under 20*. Many of these were new and underdeveloped relationships which were expected to grow in strategic importance. In simulations, failure to prioritise relationships led to organisational implosion, as internal relationships were neglected in response to the challenge of developing so many new collaborative relationships. Developing new relationships takes time and it is important to consider where that time will come from.

(2) **What kind of relationship do we want?**
The taxonomy of collaboration (Table 2.1) discussed earlier, indicates that there are real choices here. If participants have very different views of the type of relationship they are trying to develop, problems are likely to ensue. Differences of view can be accommodated, provided that they are acknowledged.

(3) **How do we expect the relationship to operate?**
People may enter into and conduct their relationships with different and untested assumptions. The frequency of meeting, the level of investment, the distribution of risk and reward are some of the practicalities of collaboration that are important to agree at the outset. Taking the time to negotiate in some detail how the relationship will operate can avoid many problems occurring later, as well as providing a benchmark for future review.

(4) **Is our experience of the relationship satisfactory?**
This question may be asked with reference to previous experience of working together where this provides the basis for some new collaborative endeavour. Or it can be asked in the context of reviewing a collaborative relationship. This can be a difficult conversation[6]. Perceptions of a relationship can vary, and a gap analysis can help crystallise the issues that need to be addressed (Dawson, 1995). Approaching this question from the perspective of the preconditions for effective relationships (see below) can provide a safe way into this conversation.

(5) **How well do organisational factors (structures, systems, processes) support the relationship?**
Chapter four highlights how poor systems can be a major risk factor, particularly with regard to supporting effective communication. Business planning cycles that are out of alignment, incompatible IT systems, different budgeting and financial control processes, and many other factors can all make it much more difficult for people to conduct effective relationships.

---

*Moreover, very often the most necessary future relationships were also currently the weakest. (Meads et al., 1999).

[6] The Harvard Negotiation Project team produced *Difficult Conversations* (Stone et al., 2000) as a guide to holding those conversations that many of us prefer to avoid if possible.

(6) **How well do 'people factors' (skills, culture) support the relationship?**
Relationships are nurtured rather than created. This means creating an
environment which will sustain the relationship (as opposed to putting it
under intolerable strain), and ensuring that both parties are able to conduct
the relationship effectively. A wide range of skills and aspects of organisational culture are relevant here. Staff have not always been selected or
promoted because of their relational skills, and some may be less naturally
inclined and able to work within a newly developed collaborative culture.

(7) **Is the relationship delivering the desired outcomes?**
This is an important check. Effective collaboration may be found in strained
relationships and not in those that achieve harmony through avoiding the
difficult but important issues. In supporting the development of new primary care organisations in England we found that highly inclusive relationships were not always effective: plenty of talk but often with difficulties in
moving to action.

One way of assessing, developing and managing relationships is to recognise
the preconditions for effective relationships[7]. This does not presuppose a particular model of a 'good' relationship: this will vary according to the context, purpose
and preferences of the participants. It does allow both parties to the relationship
to consider whether they are creating an environment which makes it easier and
more likely for an effective relationship to develop and be sustained, or whether
they are creating an inhospitable climate for effective relationships. These preconditions do not, of course, guarantee an effective relationship. They are necessary,
but not sufficient conditions. Our work in health and social care suggests five
such conditions.

Directness

Directness influences the quality of communication in the relationship. The
medium of communication affects the amount and quality of information ex-
changed. Face-to-face communication, for example, allows non-verbal signals to
be picked up and immediate responses to be made, so enabling better understanding. It is, perhaps, of particular importance around difficult or particularly
important issues. It is, however, resource intensive so it is important to ensure that
the right medium is used at the right time.

The channel of communication influences both the quality and efficiency of
information exchange. Both can be reduced if channels are blocked or if information and decisions are too often received second-hand, via messages or through
several levels of bureaucracy. Accessibility and responsiveness are key issues
here. Communication style and skills are also significant. The structure of the
communication must be complemented by the right behaviour. For instance,

---

[7] This was first set out by Schluter and Lee (1993) and applied in health care contexts in Meads *et al.*,
(1999). For current information on the availability of tools see www.relationshipsfoundation.org

a lack of openness can impede trust and undermine partnership. A cycle operates here: openness can create trust, and trust can encourage openness, but a downward spiral of decreased trust and impaired communication can also develop.

Continuity

Time can be seen as the currency of relationships. The length and stability of the relationship over time creates the opportunity for individual rapport and improved mutual understanding to develop, as well as providing a context for long-term issues to be addressed at an organisational level. Where staff turnover is high, locking in the benefits of individual and informal relationships to create an organisational history and overview of the relationship is often important. Managing change in the relationship is important if such benefits of change as career progression and bringing in new people are to be achieved without undermining the quality and effectiveness of existing relationships.

Multiplexity

Multiplexity looks at the breadth of the relationship. This can enhance mutual understanding and enable a broader appreciation of the range of skills and experience that individuals or organisations can contribute. It helps avoid strategies which ignore the realities of the underlying relationships and may open up new opportunities that arise from unsuspected common ground or unrecognised resources. Knowledge of a counterpart's organisation or agency is important in appreciating the constraints under which they work, to identify shared objectives and to develop appropriate ways of joint working. Knowledge of role or skills is important for the effectiveness of joint work and helps avoid flawed assumptions or misunderstandings, missed opportunities or suboptimal resource utilisation. Knowledge of the person (such as his or her interests or values) can strengthen the relationship and aid its management.

Parity

At times, as those working in social care, particularly, will know, it is hard to find anyone who believes they have power in a relationship. Parity does not mean equality in a relationship. Authority, influence or rewards in a relationship may rightly vary, though it is important that differentials are accepted and not abused. It is rarely a simple picture, for there are many different kinds of power (financial control, regulatory or sapiential authority, political influence, control of delivery, or exit and veto rights) in a relationship, and different parties in a relationship are likely to have different kinds of power.

Parity requires, and is fostered by, participation and involvement which ensures that people have some real say in decisions which affect their work. Lack of participation may mean that strategic objectives are not owned, may reduce morale and stifle innovation. Inadequate influence in a relationship with respect to tasks or responsibilities is a frequent source of frustration. The fairness of benefits in a relationship can engender cooperation and foster commitment to a relationship from which both parties can benefit. Fair conduct in the relationship is necessary for trust and respect. We have found that this is often cited by people whose experience of interprofessional relationships has not always been characterised by mutual respect, as a major obstacle to effective collaboration. Double standards, prejudice and favouritism are extremely corrosive.

Commonality

Commonality enables individuals and organisations to work together towards shared goals. While tensions can be creative, and there may be differences in roles and responsibilities, if these are not set in the context of some shared objectives and understanding, then the likelihood of performance-hindering conflict may be increased. Common objectives provide the basis for working together. Without real, shared and defined objectives (as opposed to generalised goals), organisations or teams may end up pulling in different directions or come into conflict over priorities. Agreement over the means of achieving goals may be as important as agreement about the goals themselves. The process by which agreement on objectives is reached is important in building commonality.

Shared culture reduces the risk of misunderstandings, the difficulty in articulating shared objectives and the lack of a shared basis for resolving differences of opinion. This applies equally to both professional and organisational cultures. A sense of common identity, of ultimately being in the same boat, can reflect the strength of the relationship as well as providing a basis for its development. This may be expressed through establishing some common culture or through developing working practices which take account of different cultures rather than just working round them or simply ignoring them. Commonality does not require uniformity. Differences can add value to a relationship, although it is important that they are seen as enriching the relationship and not just as obstacles to be overcome. The way in which disagreements are handled is also important: their resolution can strengthen commonality or may only seek to reinforce the differences.

The dividends of collaboration

Effective collaboration is rooted in compelling reasons. While it is often possible to identify win-win opportunities (and a presumption of altruism has been shown to be an inadequate basis for effective collaboration)[8], these can still require time,

---

[8] See Hudson (1998), the most authoritative writer in the UK on collaborative social care practice.

effort, investment of resources and some subordination of goals to the wider common purpose. Where collaboration does not come naturally or easily a clearly articulated dividend which can be realised early in the process helps. Conversely, collaboration which involves extra effort and hassle, and which diverts time from other important activities without adequately recognised compensating improvements in performance, is hard to sustain. The review of the National Service Framework (NSF) for cancer in the UK, for example, suggested that the scarce resource of radiographers' time is not always best invested in team meetings if that diverts the time they can give to screening activities (Commission for Health Improvement, 2001). The dividends of collaboration must also be effectively communicated. It cannot be assumed that all parties will immediately recognise them. Many people enter into collaborative relationships suspiciously and with reluctance, not least because they may already be overwhelmed with demands on their time.

The dividends of collaboration may be externally driven, reflecting the rewards for collaborative success or the costs and sanctions for collaborative failure. They may also be more internally directed, arising from the individual's sense of vocation or sources of satisfaction. The rationale for collaboration can be expressed in a number of ways. These can be grouped into those associated with the desire or requirement to seek improved quality of care, developmental concerns (which may be personal, professional, organisational or community), and the economic case for collaboration. These dividends are interlinked. Development, for example, may improve quality and this may have economic benefits. All of these are in some way an expression of the modernising trends and forces described in the previous chapter (pp. 7–11). Here, however, we are more concerned with their individual expression: how do these forces create a compelling case for someone to collaborate with others?

Collaborating to improve public health and the quality of health care

A wider definition of well-being and of the (social) determinants of health requires the contribution of a range of organisations and professions. Public health therefore requires collaboration to bring together the range of organisations and professions who have the skills, resources and opportunities to make a

Table 2.2 Cases for collaboration.

Quality	Development	Economic/market
• Promoting public health • Improving clinical care • Meeting regulatory requirements	• Personal development and satisfaction • Equipping and enabling others • Social inclusion • Organisational development in context of strategic uncertainty	• Responding to choice • Resource utilisation • Demand management

comprehensive and integrated response. A failure to collaborate effectively can represent a failure to harness all the available resources. Primary care teams, public health networks, social care providers, management teams, acute (hospital) trusts, housing providers, environmental health teams, voluntary sector organisations and user groups were all identified as key collaborative partners in a project looking at the relationships required to support the emerging public health function in newly forming primary care trusts in London (Shaw & Ashcroft, 2002).

Collaboration can improve clinical outcomes. One benefit is reducing delays in diagnosis in treatment. Trolley waits in accident and emergency departments, or delayed diagnosis and treatment of cancer and coronary heart disease may impact on clinical outcomes. While investment may be part of the solution to this, it will often be coupled with demands to redesign patient pathways and modernise service delivery. The process of identifying possible improvements, as well as the ongoing delivery of redesigned services will typically require many collaborative relationships. Collaboration is, perhaps, of particular importance for those people, for example frail elderly people, who often present with complex inter-related problems. Medicines interact. Balancing and managing care for different conditions requires effective collaboration between clinical specialisms. This can literally be a matter of life or death. Chapter four highlights the risks of failure to collaborate effectively while Chapter five looks in more detail at the importance of collaboration for maintaining and improving performance.

Collaboration for personal, professional, organisational and community development

The development case for collaboration sees it as being about growth, equipping and enabling. This is the focus of Chapter six. The focus of development may be the individual practitioners, services, organisations, or communities, with collaboration seen as supporting the exchange of skills, knowledge and opportunity.

The response of general practitioners in what were considered leading primary care organisations in the UK to the collaborative demands of partnership working around public health in the late 1990s was revealing (Meads et al., 1999). Some saw collaborative relationships as a resource and opportunity, enabling a broader role. This role was usually rooted in an ethically driven commitment to improving the public health of local communities. Some, however, saw the prospect of multiple collaborative relationships as an additional burden, complicating a more narrowly conceived medical role. Collaboration may be personally satisfying if it means seeing a client/patient's needs satisfactorily addressed even though an individual does not have sole power to achieve this. Conversely it can be very difficult continually to see the consequences of other services' failures when the capacity to influence them is limited. Collaboration can, however, open up the danger of 'mission creep': getting involved in other areas with consequential demands on time and potential loss of focus. Although awareness of this separation can also be a driver for collaboration (Huxham, 1996).

From a management perspective collaboration can be regarded as offering strategic advantages. The economic implications of this are considered later in this chapter, but first we wish to note the prospect of collaborative relationships supporting organisational stability and continuity in the context of rapid policy and organisational change. Rapid and frequent change can undermine collaboration, destroying the necessary continuity of relationships and making people reluctant to invest in relationships of limited duration. In practice, however, many of the same people remain in the system albeit with new job titles, in new organisations, and working to different policies. It is often the abiding quality of key interpersonal relationships that sustains services through such organisational change. Indeed, in such a context, investment in relationships can be seen as a key strategy for minimising personal and organisational risk and allowing development to continue.

Within the UK context there has, perhaps, historically been less of an emphasis on collaboration as a mechanism for community empowerment and development. The greater emphasis in recent years on serving excluded communities means that there are examples of this, but it is still far from being the mainstream of health and social care delivery. The agenda of personal, professional and organisational development is still much more evident.

The market and economic case for collaboration

Collaboration can be seen as a means of fostering optimal resource utilisation characterised by greater flexibility, less duplication and reduced administrative costs. This may involve professional substitution: for example, 'cheaper' nurses taking on some GP roles and therefore requiring collaboration between them (see Chapter three pp. 42–45). There are also economic aspects of the clinical case: for example, reduced hospitalisation or readmission of elderly people. The influence of the Treasury in the UK on public service reform emphasises the link between investment and demonstrable improvement. Collaboration is, therefore, required to increase the total size of the pot as well as to access different organisations' resources.

Consumer desire for convenience and quality leads to demands for greater integration of care and services. Ensuring all outpatients' tests are completed in one visit rather than over several is one simple practical example. Achieving this requires a redesign of services, and the relationships that underpin them. This is, of course, not simply a matter of convenience. There may also be significant clinical dividends as well.

Dealing with difference

Collaboration is rooted in the need to come together to access inputs, combine outputs and negotiate goals around a range of health and social care functions including, for example, health policy and planning, resourcing, improving health care (through both review and regulation) and, or course, service delivery. In order to make sense of concepts of collaboration it is important to understand the nature of the differences which give rise to the need for some collaborative coming together. These include different professional identities and cultures; different skills; different parts of the care process; differences in power, capacity and resources; and different goals and accountability.

Different health professions are, in part, a product of history but also socialise their members in different ways and may, at times, work with different theories and constructs. Individuals and organisations may have different contributions to make in the light of their varying capacity and resources. This goes beyond skills and financial resources to include, for example, access to hard-to-reach groups of people and community legitimacy, which may be a distinctive strength of, for example, voluntary sector organisations. Whilst collaboration will need to articulate common goals, this does not mean complete coherence of goals and accountability. Behind the overall shared commitment of working for patients there may be some quite divergent organisational and personal priorities. These may reflect the divergent demands of different accountabilities where the strategic collaboration to resolve these potential differences is inadequate. There have been complaints that targets in the UK, for example, have not always been consistent and the demands on social services departments to meet child protection targets have in some cases diverted resources from collaborative approaches to health care for older people. Collaboration does not remove these underlying differences. It does, however, represent both a strategy and a forum for dealing with them.

Difference can give rise to conflict. The Thomas-Kilmann conflict resolution model sees collaboration as a positive mode which can be distinguished from competing, compromising, accommodating or avoiding[9]. This can be summarised in a matrix with the two axes describing the degree of assertiveness in the relationship and the degree of cooperation. Effective collaboration requires the ability to make tough and difficult decisions: it should not be a device for avoiding them.

Collaboration is aided by the presence of some unifying force or focal point. Options include the patient or community, shared accountability or governance, service frameworks or standards, commissioning, or a common enemy. Several may be operational in any given context. What is important to note here is that both the rationale for collaboration, and the nature of the collaborative relationships involved, may differ according to the forces or factors that drive and focus that collaboration. It becomes problematic if an individual or organisation is simultaneously being encouraged to develop quite different types of relationship. This is a frequent popular criticism in the post-1997 NHS modernisation era. In the concluding section of this chapter we will therefore consider the implications

---

[9] The Thomas-Kilmann Conflict Mode Instrument (TKI) is a widely used consulting tool (Thomas & Kilmann, 1989).

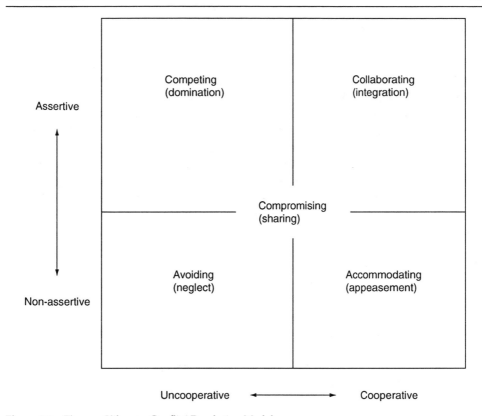

Figure 2.1 Thomas-Kilmann Conflict Resolution Model.

of focusing collaboration for the key relationships that are the concern of this book.

Focusing collaboration: implications for key relationships

The collaborative professional

Collaboration is, in part, a personal decision and is as much about who the individual is as about what they do. The professions can be the focus of collaboration, or a continuing source of difference. What, then, does the case for collaboration mean for our understanding of what it is to be a health or social care professional, and the nature of the relationship with members of the same and other professions? Implications include a shift to professionalism (Fisher, 1999), new concepts of professional identity, and new relationships of professions to other professions, partners, policy actors, the public and patients. This is seen in changes to professional regulation and registration, training and education, employment contracts, concepts and location of leadership in public services, service design and delivery, and models of the therapeutic relationship.

The differences which give rise to the need to collaborate can be subsumed under a shared identity rooted in the recognition of participation in a shared endeavour. Professional identity is not fixed and immutable. It is a product of history and culture, and will continue to develop in the light of the global modernising forces summarised in the previous chapter. While the status, identity and interrelationships of health professions may vary widely in different countries, a number of common themes can be identified which both give substance to the nature of collaboration and illustrate the different possible responses to the demands for collaboration. These are reviewed in more detail in Chapter seven, where the lessons for individual professions from this book are drawn together.

(1) **Identity**

Historically the emergence of professions can be seen in terms of the desire to establish and maintain specialised identity and status. This involved difference from the public (becoming a professional class), difference from other sectors and differentiation within sectors. The latter may be technologically driven where this requires increased specialisation, functionally driven where distinct roles develop (for example, between health visitors and district nurses), or it can be educationally driven, with different processes for training and accreditation.

Collaboration can be viewed as enabling distinct specialist professional identities to be maintained. Boundaries can be seen as points of connection rather than separation. Collaboration can be used to legitimate those boundaries by demonstrating that they do not limit health and social care, but rather enhance it by enabling a greater degree of specialisation (and the improvements in quality this can offer) than generalists could normally achieve. Alternatively collaboration can be seen as an attempt to restrict boundaries and differences. Chapter three considers equality as one of the guiding principles for health and social care relationships. In Chile this means restricting pay differentials within the primary health care team (p. 43). Where patients and communities relate more to an organisation or a service, as opposed to an individual professional, the collaborative corporate identity may become more dominant.

(2) **Influence**

One objective of grouping together is to increase influence. Professions can function as 'unions', seeking to influence pay, conditions and the work environment, as well as being some of the mechanisms through which individual practitioners can influence the policy and organisational agenda. The costs and benefits of collaboration, in terms of influence, can be hard to quantify. Constitutional arguments within the European Union provide an interesting analogy, with considerable disagreement as to whether 'pooled sovereignty' increases or reduces influence. The desire for influence may undermine collaboration if, nationally, one profession is seen to seek a position of influence at the expense of others. Collaboration can, however, extend influence: joint statements and initiatives, for example, can clearly communicate a broad-based concern which deserves to be taken seriously[10].

(3) **Independence**

Professional autonomy has been jealously guarded, and self-regulation is an important aspect of professional identity. This is increasingly seen as an earned licence, with government reserving the right to intervene to protect the public and ensure standards if necessary. Multiple accountabilities are, however, necessary to maintain the full range of checks and balances in any system. Unaccountable autonomy and controlled dependence are both dangerous. To the extent that collaboration presupposes difference it can be seen as protecting the independent legitimacy which may be needed if, for example, the political process loses legitimacy and public confidence. Competing claims to advocacy of the public interest can be destabilising, but a collaborative integration of different accountabilities is a source of strength.

(4) **Improvement**

There is a strong scientific tradition of seeking improvement in health care through medical research. The culture of improvement through research into improved collaborative care practices is less deeply rooted. Nursing can perhaps be seen as more open to this as, historically, the nursing profession has been less involved in medical research and nursing skills, and more closely linked to working practice than to medical technology. If quality can be regained as a positive concept, rather than a suspect instrument of control, then this aspect of professional culture should be a positive force for collaboration.

(5) **Income**

The desire to narrow or maintain pay differentials should not be underestimated as a factor influencing attitudes. Where collaboration narrows role boundaries, differentials may become harder to maintain, as is the case in Chile. A shift from hierarchical to team relationships also influences attitudes to differentials. Pay is a key indicator of recognition and status and where collaboration starts to impinge on this it may be seen as more threatening.

Partners

The promotion of partnerships by modernising policies and health promoting strategies in the UK has given a structural focus to collaboration. These new

---

[10] An example of an interprofessional statement is that issued in 2002 by the Royal College of Psychiatrists and the Law Society to convey the concerns of both professions about proposed reforms to the Mental Health Act. The statement can be found at http://www.rcpsych.ac.uk/press/preleases/pr/pr_336.htm

organisational relationships provide the context for new professional relationships. Examples of this can be seen at different levels. In England, since 2000,
Local Strategic Partnerships (LSPs) have been created as a focus for inter-agency
coordination and collaboration focused on local authority areas[11]. Some seek
to provide strong local strategic leadership, integrating budgets and enabling
agencies to work together on agreed strategic priorities. Others remain little more
than a forum for communication. In some ways they mirror the previous development pattern of NHS primary care groups, with a number of different relationship
styles emerging in the context of local uncertainty (at least in some areas) as to
whether a given structure will prove to be the real focus of collaboration[12].

There is also, in the UK, a plethora of delivery partnerships including, for
example, teenage pregnancy, smoking cessation, mental health, drugs, child
protection, Sure Start, Connexions and many others. With some public health
professionals participating in up to ten partnerships, this leads to concern about
partnership fatigue, the need to rationalise partnerships and a desire to see
'evidence-based relationships'. These partnerships may emerge as a result of
wider strategic collaboration; be driven in response to policy, targets and funding
streams; or be built on a longer history of operational collaboration. The formal
establishment of a partnership is usually intended to remove structural barriers. It
provides a mechanism for financial implications of collaboration to be dealt with
and should enable joint working to be more closely integrated with participating
organisations' own strategy and planning. While a structural focus for collaboration is helpful, it is important that this reflects an underlying strategic focus. Too
often, in the past, the NHS has changed structures to the detriment of the
underlying relationships which are needed to sustain their effective contribution
to promoting health and delivering services.

Policy

The following chapter illustrates how different policy themes can lead to quite
different examples of collaboration, influencing the context for collaboration as
well as introducing or minimising barriers to collaboration. Each of the potential
focal points for collaboration can be promoted and encouraged through policy.
Here, we are concerned with the ways in which the policy process itself can be a
focus for collaboration. Effective collaboration requires 'joined-up' policy, the
making of which is a collaborative endeavour, not just between departments
but also between civil servants and practitioners. In the UK, recently, the Cabinet
Office has sought to encourage a more systems-based approach to policy[13]. The

---

[11] The policy context for LSPs is neighbourhood renewal (Social Exclusion Unit 2001). Details about
LSP structure can be found in DETR (2001).
[12] Meads and Ashcroft (2000) describe the ambivalence of health professions towards the modernising
reforms of the late 1990s.
[13] The Performance and Innovation Unit, now absorbed within the Strategy Unit in the UK Cabinet
Office, produced a number of reports and discussion papers about improving the policy making
process of which PIU (2000) is an example.

recognition that policy cannot directly control outcomes suggests a more collaborative self-regulating approach. Government is to be seen as part of the system and not the external mechanic or driver. Pragmatic politics ('what counts is what works') emphasises the roles of pilots and beacons in what has become 'a culture of audited experimentation' (Kay, 2003). In such a context policy is not just an external force to which health professionals are obliged to respond. Rather they can (if recognised as successful exponents of innovative best practice) become partners in a reforming process.

That, of course, presumes an underlying shared goal. The reality is ambivalence. The sense of being trusted partners in policy is, at best, elusive. In policy the shift from collaboration to conflict is very easy. This may be seen in Government itself. In England, Public Service Agreements imply collaboration between Treasury (funder) and spending Government ministries (providing, commissioning and managing), with policy portrayed as collaboration between investment and reform or modernisation. The experience of this may suggest perceptions of conflicting control and accountability rather than collaboration.

Public

Organisations and professions all relate to the public. This basic shared duty of service and accountability can become the focus for strategic collaboration. This, of course, depends on whether the individual relationships with the public are construed in the same way and whether the shared relationship with the public is a stronger unifying force than other more divisive forces which may be shaping the health care system. In the UK context, community involvement tends to be seen as a public health and management responsibility. 'User' involvement in services tends to be more focused on individual patients than communities.

Collaboration here is concerned with local strategy, legitimacy and accountability. Despite some good local and international examples of community involvement this is proving difficult in the UK. The post-1997 Health Improvement Plans did not really engage the public. Community Health Councils are being replaced. Local Strategic Partnerships are still principally a forum for organisational relationships rather than local democratic or professional engagement. In 2004 there is still scepticism about whether Foundation Hospitals will be genuinely community owned mutual organisations. 'Lay' membership of the board cannot, on its own, change a centralised political culture where local elections are often characterised by very low turn-outs and voter apathy. Voluntary organisations and community groups may act as a proxy for more broadly based community involvement. However, in a project with London PCTs we discovered many difficulties in relating with a fragmented and under-resourced voluntary sector (Shaw & Ashcroft, 2002). Knowing who to involve, and how to invest in their capacity to be an effective partner without compromising their ability to resource their core activities proved a challenge.

Patients

Health care can be seen as a collaborative endeavour between individual patients, their relatives (or other carers and advocates), and health care professionals. Empowered patients can serve as a focal point for collaboration, but not always. They may be able to achieve this through the ways in which they purchase care, through acting as an administrative safety net, or by being the most reliable mechanism for exchanging information. This is, of course, easiest for the articulate, confident, knowledgeable and well-resourced patient. For those who are seriously ill with no relatives or other advocates, who do not have ready access to a phone, who are frightened or confused, and who are not sure what they can reasonably expect, such a role is unrealistic. They may hope that others will practice 'patient-centred' care, focusing their collaborative endeavours around them, but they cannot themselves exert the gravitational force to pull the collaborative endeavour together. The potential for the patient to act as a focus for collaboration will also be influenced by different models of the therapeutic relationship. The more the patient is viewed as a partner in the care process, the greater the likelihood that they can influence collaborative behaviour.

Lessons

The case for collaboration is, in part, the necessary response to key policy themes. There are also real dividends for professions, patients and organisations (see Chapter five for a more in depth examination of the links between collaboration and performance). Collaboration is a rational choice, although we may not always be aware of our part in a collaborative process. Chapter four explores how the frail reality of collaboration in the hurried note or phone call can easily break down. The case for collaboration does not, of course, always seem clear cut: nor is the practice easy. Collaboration can be difficult and costly. Like all relationships it demands continuing investment. At one of our workshops in 1999 the plea of one public health worker, convinced of the case for collaboration but overwhelmed with the demands of many partnerships, was eloquent: 'How can I know what investment in which relationships is worthwhile?'

We cannot, here, provide a complete guide to 'evidence-based relationships' but we can distil a number of lessons. In specific contexts we would want to be more precise about the kinds of relationships that could (or should) be pursued. There are, however, benefits in the broad field of meaning that we have retained in using the term 'collaboration'. For those who are feeling their way into more collaborative ways of working it may be helpful to know that there are options. The taxonomy of collaboration set out in Table 2.1 is not a menu, but may suggest aspects of collaboration that are attainable. Collaboration is aided by thinking strategically about how to achieve what is important for the individual, and for those to whom they are accountable. In practice this means clear (preferably shared) decisions about which are the most important relationships, what kinds of collaboration will be pursued, and what dividends can be realised.

Doing this requires acknowledging differences and identifying unifying factors. Here, collaboration becomes personal. The demand for collaboration, expressed in policy themes but rooted in health and social care needs, may be inescapable: its practice requires commitment, generosity[14] and change. Collaboration means rethinking who you are and what you seek to do: this is the context for effective changes to structures and working practices. Differences and identities are re-focused in the light of common purpose: the demand by policy, patients and the public for accountable service. This light may be refracted into different roles and contributions, but these can no longer sustain an isolated existence.

The final lesson is to own this agenda. It is inescapable. It can be imposed, although not so effectively. That is the negative case for collaboration. Positively, owning the agenda is about fulfilment and development. It is the route to quality. It is the means of personal, professional, organisational and community development. It creates opportunities and accesses resources. It restores confidence and legitimacy. An old Zulu proverb says that, 'You are only a person because of other people.' That is true for professions today.

Conclusion

Collaboration is about working together in the face of both commonality and difference. It can be described in many ways, including its goals, its structural context and the level within that structure, the processes involved, the use of power, the proximity of the participants, and its duration and complexity. Developing collaborative relationships is aided by strategic clarity about the relationships and by creating an environment that sustains them. Clearly identified attainable benefits encourage collaboration. These dividends of collaboration can be summarised in terms of quality, enabling development and economic benefits. Collaboration also requires some unifying factor. Each of the six key relationships of the modern professional has a part to play in this. However, while there are many powerful forces which make the demand for collaboration inescapable, it is most likely to succeed if the agenda is owned. Collaboration is as much about who the individual is as what they do.

Bibliography

Commission for Health Improvement (2001) *NHS Cancer Care in England and Wales: National Service Framework Assessments No. 1.* Commission for Health Improvement, London.

---

[14] The case for the importance of generosity made by Iles (1997) remains both powerful and relevant.

Dawson, S. (1995) *Analysing Organisations*. Macmillan, Basingstoke.

Department of the Environment, Transport and the Regions (2001) *Local Strategic Partnerships: Government Guidance March 2001*. Department of the Environment, Transport and the Regions, London.

Estlund, C. (2003) *Working Together: How Workplace Bonds Strengthen a Diverse Democracy*. OUP, Oxford.

Fisher, E. (1999) *Professionalism and Expertise in the Public Services: a Historical and Conceptual Overview*. University of Southampton, Southampton.

Haggerty, J., Reid, R., Freeman, G. *et al.*, (2003) Continuity of care: a multidisciplinary review. *British Medical Journal*, **27**, 22 November, p. 1219.

Hudson, R. (1998) *Primary Care and Social Care*. Nuffield Institute, Leeds.

Huxham, C. (1996) Collaboration and collaborative advantage. In: *Creating Collaborative Advantage*. (ed. C. Huxham), pp 1–18. Sage, London.

Iles, V. (1997) *Really Managing Health Care*. Open University Press, Buckingham.

Kay, J. (2003) *The Truth about Markets: their Genius, their Limits, their Follies*. Allen Lane, London.

Meads, G., Killoran, A., Ashcroft, J. & Cornish, Y. (1999) *Mixing Oil and Water*. HEA Publications, London.

Meads, G. & Ashcroft, J. (2000) *Relationships in the NHS*. RSM Press, London.

Nash, V. (2002) *Reclaiming Community*. IPPR, London.

Performance and Innovation Unit (PIU) (2000) *Wiring It Up: Whitehall's Management of Cross-Cutting Policies and Services*. Cabinet Office, London.

Schluter, M. & Lee, D. (1993) *The R Factor*. Hodder & Stoughton, London.

Shaw, S. & Ashcroft, J. (2002) *The Impact of Primary Care Trusts' Emerging Relationships on the Public Health Function*. Department of General Practice and Primary Care, Queen Mary's School of Medicine and Dentistry, London.

Shaw, S., Taylor, S. & Petchey, R. (2002) *Primary Care Trusts and the Public Health Function: Final report*. Health Services Research Unit, Queen Mary's School of Medicine and Dentistry, University of London, London.

Social Exclusion Unit (2001) *A New Commitment to Urban Renewal: National Strategy Action Plan*. Department for Transport, Local Government and the Regions, London.

Stone, D., Patton, B., & Heen, S. (2000) *Difficult Conversations: How to Discuss What Matters Most*. Penguin, New York.

Thomas, K. & Kilmann, R. (1989) *The Thomas-Kilmann Conflict Mode Instrument*. Xicom, Tuxedo, New York.

Wilkinson, D. & Appelbee, E. (1999) *Implementing Holistic Government: Joined-up action on the ground*. Policy Press, Bristol.

Further Reading

Active Community Unit (1998) *Compact on Relations between Government and the Voluntary and Community Sector in England*. Home Office, London.

Ashcroft, J. (2001) Releasing the Dividends of New Partnerships. In: *Trust in Experience: Transferable Learning for Primary Care Trusts*. (eds G. Meads & P. Meads), pp. 49–68. Radcliffe Medical Press, Abingdon.

Barnes, M., Sullivan, H., & Matka, E., (2001) *Building Capacity for Collaboration: The National Evaluation of Health Action Zones*. University of Birmingham, Birmingham.

Loxley, A. (1997) *Collaboration in Health and Welfare: Working with Difference.* Jessica Kingsley
    Publishers, London.
Neighbourhood Renewal Unit (2002) *Collaboration and Coordination in Area-Based Initiatives.*
    Department for Transport, Local Government and the Regions, London.
Sullivan, T. (1998) *Collaboration, a Health Care Imperative.* McGraw-Hill, New York.

3 The Case For

Perspective

It is now time to broaden our horizons. The last chapter has provided a range
of models of collaboration drawn from, and directed at, the daily operational
practice and local organisation of health and social care. Many of these
are derived from developments within the UK, where collaboration has been
fundamental to the drafting and delivery of the Government's millennium NHS
Plan. In this chapter the theories and concepts which shape policy come from
further afield. Our perspective is global. The ideas we will examine are
those which transcend national boundaries in both their impact on professional
behaviour and their relationship with the immediate issues and local settings of
health and social care. Professionals often do not like change, and sometimes for
very good reasons. But the kinds of ideas contained in this chapter are those that
help make up some of the trends in what is often called 'globalisation', and there
are very few professionals who would not recognise the very real impact of
this term.

The doctor, nurse or therapist only has to turn on his or her computer in a
consultation to see that the sources of information and advice available can now
come directly from any location. The number, role, structure and combination of
specialist health professions themselves all have to adjust to the radical pressures
of this globalisation. Some contemporary commentators have even gone so far as
to suggest that the traditional concept of professions in health care is in jeopardy,
as increasingly we relate to those who provide our clinical services via the
managing host organisation rather than through the profession itself[1]. What is
certain is that the world is changing and that the next generation of those
practising in the health and social services need to collaborate to understand the
nature and implications of globalising developments and how best to respond to
them. While historically most health professions have been global in nomencla-
ture and outlook, membership of international associations and overseas conference attendance is no longer enough.

---

[1] See, for example, Exworthy and Halford (1999) on the impact of the 'New Managerialism', which
was originally critiqued by Harrison and Pollitt (1994).

Purpose

The aim, accordingly, of the next few pages is to choose and illustrate key policy ideas which are of fundamental and universal relevance to modern professional relationships. Employing our sixfold framework for these relationships, as described earlier in Chapter one (pp. 6–7), we will consider a set of basic health principles with some of their modern interpretations, drawing on the global literature under each heading. All of the supporting concepts for these legitimising principles have been selected in order to strike a chord, chiming with the actual experience of practitioners. To reinforce this effect in each case a country has also been identified as a 'beacon site' example for the kinds of collaboration that express in action the selected ideas. These examples have been drawn largely from the recent international research programme referred to in Table 1.1 (p. 6). In this programme we have examined some of those countries which have explicitly applied 'modernising' policy frameworks, in the pursuit of profound partnership based reforms in their health and social care systems. Table 3.1 sets out the list of global theories and concepts, derived from the frameworks in our study and from the relevant supporting literature, used in this chapter and their country case examples.

This particular framework of 'globalisation' reflects the recent impetus given to collaborative ventures by organisations with international and continental responsibilities for health policy steerage. Globally, in such agencies as the World Bank, DFID (UK) and the WHO, there has been a growing level of anxiety at what are perceived to be increased levels of institutional inertia, especially in countries overwhelmingly dependent on single sources of public funding and accountability (e.g. Switzerland, UK). In many areas of health care need – from capital infrastructure investment to major vaccination programmes – decisive responses have been almost exclusively dependent on innovative partnerships which extend well beyond conventional professional and political boundaries. These 'third sector' partners are distinguished by their diversity. Non-governmental organisations (NGOs) can have an enormous variety of sponsors and stakeholders in health and social care.

Table 3.1 Global policy.

Key relationship	Country example	Health principle	Associated ideas
(1) with same profession	Portugal	autonomy	complexity, participation
(2) with other professions	Chile	equity	distributional justice substitution
(3) with (new) partners	Greece	integration	transdiscipline network
(4) with policy actors	Philippines	system	learning organisation sector-wide approach
(5) with public (representatives)	Finland	quality	managed care enrichment
(6) with patients	Peru	trust	deconcentration civil society

A new hospital, for example, in Shanghai has its origins in a collaboration between politicians, bankers and doctors in the USA; while in the UK the post-2004 Diagnostic and Treatment Centres depend upon a venture capitalist company's capacity to pool spare specialist surgical capacity from the likes of Austria, Spain and Germany[2]. Contributions by private companies and academic establishments, in particular, are encouraged by international policy making forums. Especially in developed countries, health care professionals may have ideological and even ethical objections to such contributions. In the past there has been a tendency to resist or even reject the role of non-public sector organisations as either intellectually irrelevant or morally inappropriate. The intrusion of private health care companies, or community-based colleges with multidisciplinary faculties, could be seen as contaminating both for professions and the principles of publicly funded and professionally sovereign services. Of course in developing countries where, at the turn of the century, analysts still calculated that over half of health care resources were still reliant on the 'Third Sector' (Schieber & Maeda, 1999) such principles are often regarded by local doctors, nurses and welfare workers as either pretentious piety or protective capitalism. For these health professionals multiple collaborations and social solidarity go hand in hand.

In 1998 a World Health Organization report captured the essential imperative to site sustainable partnerships at the heart of health policies able to support long-term improvements, with its title: *Everybody's Business* (WHO, 1998). A decade earlier it had faced up to the chronic imbalance between public expenditure and public health requirements across Africa with its promotion, in the Bamako Initiative, of enhanced access and quality, based on user fees and co-payment mechanisms for medical and nursing care. By 1999 it was able to convene a meeting of 56 different country representatives from nation states actively developing mixed payment and multi-professional health care systems. In July of the same year the Arizona Charter was published, once again with the WHO and, in this case, UNESCO backing. It linked new partnerships in health specifically to the needs of disadvantaged groups through what it termed 'multidimensional action' and the 'catalytic role' of universities 'mobilising the various resources needed (to) facilitate the convergence of disparate interests and create coalitions among key players in governments, health professions and communities'.[3]

These words tally directly with those of other international agencies such as UNICEF, TUFH, DFID (UK) and, not least, the World Bank, which since 1993 has

---

[2] Interestingly, in the autumn of 2003 the only successful tender bids for setting up the next stage of subregional Diagnostic and Treatment Centres in England came from the private sector, reversing earlier trends of lower NHS staff and overhead costs, and indicating new levels of collaboration between capital investors and both domestic and foreign clinicians. A parallel Chinese experience is described in Walsh (1998).

[3] The Arizona Charter led to the setting up of the international Universities in Solidarity for the Health of the Disadvantaged (UNI-SOL) project, details of which can be obtained from the WHO Collaborating Center on Border and Rural Health Research, College of Medicine, The University of Arizona, 2501 East Elm Street, Tucson, Arizona 85716, USA: tel +1 (520) 626-7946, email UNISOL@rho.arizona.edu

been committed to supporting policies of fully combined economic and social development. Its *Investing in Health* report then was a watershed for future health systems development and the profile of professional relationships. Economic growth was recognised as no longer the chief precondition for health improvement. Rather the latter was seen as a legitimate object for the Bank and its global regional counterparts to invest in directly, as an economic sector in its own right, the progress of which would foster new industries, commerce and technologies. As with all such landmark global policies its local repercussions for individual professionals have often taken at least a decade to filter down and be felt. However, the Bank's twin injunction in 1993 that health care systems should be underpinned by strategies which ensured both collective self-responsibility at community levels and cost effectiveness at governmental levels, opened the door to diversity, deregulation and competition for professions across the world. In Europe, for example, Target 18 of the WHO Region relates to 'Developing Human Resources for Health' both amongst health professionals and, equally significantly, with 'professionals in other sectors' (Buchan & Dal Paz, 2002). The European Union itself promotes partnership working even more vigorously, somewhat paradoxically, because health care systems remain, under its principles of subsidiarity, the responsibility of separate nation states. In this context, collaboration is the main mechanism at its disposal, through the terms of its development grants; its allied policies for the environment, employment and economic expansion; and its statutory standards and regulations.

Of course, in genuine multinational emergencies, collaboration by health professionals with each of the six partners listed in our Chapter one frameworks (pp. 6–7) is quickly forthcoming. Witness global responses to the AIDS/HIV virus or the SARS outbreaks. At these times collaboration is the only response. The problems arise when it is the optional response. Then international partnership based policies can take a long time to reach into practice. The 1978 Alma Ata declaration on Primary Health Care is nowadays accepted with virtual unanimity. But it was not until 1993, 1994 and 2001 respectively that its 'pillar' collaborative values of community participation, inter-sectoral alliances, equity and professional partnership were formally adopted in policy by, for example, the national governments of Sri Lanka, South Africa and Thailand – three middle ranking countries well removed from the relegation zone in international health systems performance league tables. As this indicated, globalisation and the universal policy drivers it encompasses, is a thematic which affects us all, but for health professionals in different settings at varying paces and pressures.

In such circumstances it is better to be prepared. Having scanned the global environment for the organisational sources of collaborative cultural change let us now turn once more to the relationships of the modern health professionals. It is helpful to gain a better appreciation of the specific policy principles and concepts that, in the modern context of globalisation, are exercising a formative influence on practice.

With same profession

Autonomy is a relational concept for the modern health professional. In the past professional autonomy and all that goes with it – rights to self regulation, independent terms of employment, proprietorship and high social status – have been founded on assertions of exclusive knowledge, skills and experience. The claims to clinical expertise, in hierarchical structures, have defined the pecking order at ward rounds in hospitals through to the powers of prescription in general practice. Professional autonomy and organisational separation have been almost synonymous. Each health profession has had its own headquarters, codes of conduct and representative structures. Indeed the trend throughout the past century was for each profession to set its own separate direction. In the UK in 1900 there were only two approved Royal Colleges: for surgeons and physicians. In 2000 over 60 separate and Government approved national associations were operating and when the new regulatory Health Professions Council was being set up in 2002 the continuing shift to sub-specialists was illustrated by the attempt to register no fewer than seven professional titles just in podiatry. On economic cost grounds, if nothing else, it was a trend that could not be allowed to continue.

Placing professional autonomy in its modern global policy context of such key supporting ideas as *complexity* and *participation* helps effect this change. Put simply, complexity is about understanding the systems of health and social care, from the human body to the hospital institution, as interactive and multi-variable organisms, in which change often takes place in ways that are unpredictable if linear and exclusively internal approaches only are used. In this framework the cause and effect, symptoms, diagnosis and drugs based treatment and cure models of conventional medicine become outdated. Complexity itself implies that progress is made through participation: intervening as a health professional as one component of the appropriate complex of forces, both internal and external, which together can deliver efficacious outcomes. Change does not depend on variables in direct contact with each other but on factors which in aggregate may be influenced to produce the desired direction of change even though they may not appear to be in relationship to one another.[4]

The ideas of complexity and participation underpin much action research and are closely allied, as we shall see later in this chapter, to modern chaos and systems theories. For the autonomy of the health professional the two ideas come together in contemporary developments for governance. Whether clinical or corporate, governance is essentially a participative and complex form of accountability. In England, for example, its introduction in 1999 was as:

---

[4] See Griffiths & Sweeney (2001) for a specific application of Complexity Theory to general medical practice.

'a framework for bringing together all local activity for improving and assessing clinical quality into a single coherent programme, which everyone as an organisation can be part of and work towards.'

(HSC, 1999, Executive Summary, p. 3.)

Its processes are essentially interactive between the internal and external: through the various mechanisms of controls assurance, risk management and performance monitoring. These are designed to promote an effective dynamic between nationally set standards and locally driven developments. Under the terms of governance the health professional is individually *and* collectively accountable, and this accountability includes compliance with agreed organisational processes and policies. In short, health professionals become formally responsible both for each other and to a range of legitimate political interests. They must participate and autonomy is earned through their response to collective responsibility. Successful patient care becomes equated with the sum of professional collaborations in which governance mechanisms seek to harness the complexity of different contributions and their usually indirect relationships. Again, to quote a recent English policy statement:

'Governance provides a framework within which local organisations can work to improve and assure the quality of clinical services for patients. Implementing and maintaining risk management and organisational controls is fundamental to assuring the success of clinical governance, providing a solid foundation upon which to build an environment in which quality care can be provided and clinical excellence can flourish. "Getting the organisation right" will significantly increase the likelihood of achieving the desired outcomes in relation to meeting the needs of patients'.

(NHS Executive, March 1999, p. 3, para. 9.)

As this suggests, the organisation rather than the profession has become globally the pivotal unit in health and social care. The modern organisation has the scope to respond to complexity in ways that the traditionally peer based, and often rather unidimensional health profession could not. Similarly it is a forum for participation at a time when this has become a quasi-moral value recognised as an individual right in health and social care. From diagnosis to treatment, from needs assessment to commissioning: all are now fundamentally participative activities of partnership for health and social care professionals.

That this applies to new forms of collaboration within professions is highlighted by the recent Portuguese experience and the range of joint initiatives undertaken by its general medical practitioners. Portugal is particularly interesting because the doctors have reorganised themselves as a profession, with retained and strengthened autonomy, in response to the policy drivers we have discussed above, during a period when there has been a hiatus (or even a void) in health policy at Governmental level. Since 1999, in Lisbon, there has been a regular turnover of Ministers of Health and a lack of consistent strategic direction as a result. The Social Democratic Government, elected in February 2002, moved away from previous political administrations' commitments to universal public primary care services. It has focused on strengthening general management at provincial levels; reducing hospital deficits with new DRG based budgets, and introducing private finance initiatives (e.g. issuing 11 tenders in 2003). Its unit of planning is the (complex) Local Health System (LHS), the constituents of which can come from any sector, regardless of formal status. The traditionally charitable *Misericordias*, for example, are being converted into small health and social care businesses, and an LHS with 30 000 people qualifies for multi-specialist provision (e.g. obstetrics, dermatology, paediatrics), where the majority of the specialists will either be private clinic or hospital based.

The response of general medical practitioners in Portugal has been robust and rooted in new collaborations. Historically a low key, relatively low salaried status and individualistic profession their National Association (APMCG) has grown rapidly to over 4 500 members, its largest ever number. In 2003 250 of these were piloting capitation based performance related pay in areas covering a total population of 500 000 people and 280 primary care centres have taken part in quality assurance programmes. Clinical governance procedures and protocols based on smaller practice units have been adopted through the GP-led Institute for Quality in Health Care. This Institute exemplifies the new collaborations through its 75% European Union funding, and its support for community participation via the local publication of practice audits, and its proposals for service redistribution linked to the Interior Ministry's post-1996 programmes for 'Social Insertion' of disadvantaged groups. The APMCG has formed alliances with universities in Coimbra and Porto to lobby Government and has developed national post-qualifying educational curricula and criteria, and international scanning mechanisms for transferable learning.

In short, the profession in Portugal has done most of the things itself that in the UK, for example, have been required of it by national government. As a result, in both countries the role of the health professional and the shape of the health profession looks different. The former now collaborates with community, the independent and academic sectors and national agencies as part of his or her normal professional activities. These incorporate developmental, educational and managerial functions as a result. Collectively the health profession is more differentiated and graduated, with specialist functions in research, education, finance, audit and quality. But at both levels the new pattern of collaborative relationships has meant the retention and, indeed, fortification of autonomy. As our example of Portugal helps to demonstrate, professional autonomy and the integrity of the individual profession now have to be validated by successful processes of participation and the knowledge management of its complex outcomes.

With other professions

Where Portugal illustrates the need for professions to develop new relationships between their own constituents Chile is a classic contemporary example of the collaborations now required between different health professionals. In Chile, for example, health professionals belong to a single national trade union to maximise their political bargaining power with Government and other corporate players. Basic salary differentials across frontline health professions are restricted to 40%. The new model urban health centre primary care team for a population of 20 000 people, in the public service sector in 2003, had a local mix of the nationally defined standard team membership of nine professions: general medical practitioner, dentist, psychologist, social worker, nurse, midwife (matron), dispenser, physical therapist and nutritionist. All referrals are owned by the whole team, regardless of the initial point of patient contact. Back pain and depression, for instance, are equally the responsibility of the general medical practitioner, psychologist and dispenser, even if it is the nurse or the nutritionist who makes the initial preliminary diagnosis. Funding from the National Health Fund (FONASA) is now substantially (40%) based on the interprofessional unit's performance in relation to 56 (extending to 108 in 2004) Chile-wide national priority programmes (e.g. cancer, oral health) each with a preventive emphasis. Under the guiding influence of the Medical School at *La Universidad Catholica* in Santiago, generic problem-based learning (PBL) and teamwork approaches are fundamental to each health profession's training curriculum, and the new 'super-specialists' in family medicine have a minimum ten year pre-qualifying period.

The Chilean system is founded on the modern principle of *equity*, where the equitable allocation of resources is based, not on individual professions' numbers, or even the size of service units, but on health needs and outcomes assessments. Equitable health status is the overriding goal. This meaning of equity in health systems is tied to the wider public policy idea of *distributional justice*, which globally is most apparent in such countries as Brazil, South Africa and Zimbabwe, where there are extreme ranges of income. In South Africa, for example, primary health care development has been informed by a 'vertical equity' perspective in which the poorest are placed at the heart of health service decision making. This meant that South Africa was the first sub-Saharan state to withdraw from the Bamoko Agreement (p. 38) by abolishing user fees and progressively rolling out free services, beginning with pregnant women and children under six in 1994. In 2003, in Chile, the annual per capita allocation of FONASA ranged from $950 in non-poor urban areas to $1345 in rural poor regions. This difference of over 40% again is distributional justice in action, and of course in developed countries, such as the UK, ring-fenced NHS funds for access targets relating to ethnic minority and other disadvantaged sections of the population indicate that the modern understanding of equity is far from just a Third World figure of speech.

This policy interpretation of equity requires new forms of collaboration. It does not automatically respect individual professional disciplines and their past traditions. It requires value for resources. It is supported on the one hand by the concept and practice of distributional justice, and on the other by *substitution*. The two terms are complementary. Substitution amongst health professionals in Western countries is sometimes seen as a dirty word. It can have connotations of simply doing things more cheaply with a consequent loss of expertise and, possibly, power as well, for the profession being substituted. This sense of suspicion has surrounded, in particular, the emergence of nurse practitioners. It has also been evident in the UK, for example, in the local transfers of diabetic retinopathy screening services from the ophthalmologist to the optometrist; the shift of mental health advocacy from approved social workers to the NHS 'Gateway' programme and the creation of hospital alternative orthopaedic surgery production lines in new Diagnostic and Treatment Centres. Each of these changes dramatically alters the profile of costs and it is easy to understand why substitution can be viewed as simply an economic measure.[5]

An international perspective, however, makes clear that it is not. Substitution is more often and more accurately understood as an innovative response to new information and evidence; substitution gives communities the option of utilising their existing resources more efficiently and effectively. It is in this context of providing health care differently, but just as well, that we can view the 60 000 health promoters of Mexico, the 'triple trained' nurses of Uganda and several southern African states and the 1000 new practice based Graduate Mental Health Workers now being trained in England. Substitution in relation to the expanded skills mix offered by new personnel such as these should be understood not as like-for-like replacements, but rather as a soccer style, squad development, increasing the alternatives to fit the particular time and place. The Graduate Mental Health Workers, for example, came from the recognition (in the 1999 NHS National Service Framework) that with one in six people suffering from mental health problems, and local authorities spending less than 5% of their social services budgets in this area, effective community care and coordination could never come from a service confined to clinically based consultant psychiatrists and psychiatric nurses (DoH, 1999). In Mexico the Government's *Progresa* Project and the main insurance fund (IMSS) reached the same conclusion in respect of rural primary health care, which led to the new army of health promoters. Health Aids personnel in India were derived from similar local needs and outcomes assessments. Substitution is very often the vehicle for distributional justice in terms of seeking to ensure equity of health status across disparate locations.

For health professionals the impact is many more collaborations. There are emerging health professions, often with their roots in traditional (Chinese) medicine and healing, such as the authorised *Yatiri* healers in Bolivia. There are semi-professions which draw on knowledge from across past professions – such as the Graduate Mental Health Workers. There are those whose roles emerge from within local community networks and social structures, like the Health Aids and Promoters cited above, or the Health Technicians of Costa Rica. And then there is the realignment taking place within established professions with, for example, the conversion of Internists to General Medical Practitioners in such countries as Slovakia and Lithuania and, led by the USA, the restructuring of

---

[5] A case study detailing the attitudinal dilemmas that require sensitive management, arising from professional substitutions, and relating to new optometric developments is contained in our earlier work: Meads (1999).

nursing into at least five types, each with its own specialisms and grading structures (Buchan & Dal Paz, 2002).

In Chile, remarkably, the pursuit of equity through new collaborative arrangements for its health care professions has led to a major shift in public support for the public services. Despite a strong economy, levels of individual subscription to the consortium of private health insurers (ISAPRES) fell from a peak of 4.1 million in 1997 to 2.9 million in 2003. The number of ISAPRES has been halved to 14. Across the country local mayors have begun to make significant contributions to the new multi-professional services sometimes 'substituting' some of their own staff to health centres and their outposts. At the Catholic University the Dean has an apposite phrase for describing those doctors who fail to recognise the changing world of new interprofessional relationships, and their own retraining needs. 'They have mud feet', he says. He is right. Equity is the level playing field for health and social care in the twenty-first century, on which the professionals that collaborate successfully will be those ready to share power and expertise with each other, redistribute resources and tailor their responses to particular needs.

With new partners

Equity, of course, rose to prominence in health policies of the late twentieth century as an essentially economic concept during the period of 'marketisation'. The pursuit of equitable resource allocations was regarded as an important prerequisite for effectively and efficiently (re-) balancing health care supply and demand. It led to the development of such purchasing agencies as Health Maintenance Organisations (in the USA), General Practice Fund holders (in the UK) and Sickness Funds (in the Netherlands), utilising the techniques of managed care. Nowadays, the buzz word is *integration*. Again it is derived principally from the economic perspectives which, over the past decade, have continued to dominate the global literature on health systems development.[6]

Integration, like equity, sounds good. It is a pleasing word; it can be applied readily and easily to services, organisations and even to the patient experience itself. But health and social care professionals are, nevertheless, wary of its too frequent and, perhaps, too facile applications. Integration can be a euphemism: the word that requires a sharing of resources when the real issue is maintaining high clinical (and costly) skills: the word that leads to mergers and structural solutions when the real issues are respecting different traditions, separate cultures and vocational service commitments.

Equity recovered its integrity as a value by being attached to health status, critically supported by such public policy principles as those of distributional

---

[6] The Bibliography provides examples of this literature with Lassey *et al.* offering a typical global typology of emerging integrated delivery systems as part of what they see as the global trend of 'managed competition' (Lassey *et al.*, 1997, pp. 318–50).

justice and substitution. This has led to the kinds of collaborations between health professions we discussed in the previous section. In the same way, properly supported, the pursuit of integration can and does pave the way for positive, exciting and productive new partnerships. Most obviously this is apparent in the different fields of health services research. Such research may be clinical and/or non-clinical. It is founded on what some Colombian Medical Schools have described as: 'Research as *transdiscipline*'. With this idea of knowledge management comes power and influence. Applying management to knowledge for such purposes means scanning the intellectual horizons across the physical and social sciences; harnessing quantitative and qualitative data and, above all, utilising relevant intelligence regardless of whether it comes from a multinational life science company or an academic website.

In Colombia the new partnerships forged by health professionals, remarkably for a developing country, took the level of overall expenditure on health care to over 10% of GDP in 2001. This was at a time when less than half of the country's 43 million population were eligible for the benefits of the post-1993 Compulsory Health Plan (POS) through membership of one of the approved national insurance programmes. These new partnerships have been many and varied, with a truly 'modern' profile of novel collaborations for local doctors, nurses and welfare workers arising from the decentralisation laws of 1990 and 1993 (Laws 10 and 60; Bossert, 1998; Pan American Health Organisation, 2002). For example, these include poor areas' local private health cooperatives or *Empresas Solidarias de Salud* (ESS), which can contract with both communities and commercial companies. They have collaborated with health professionals to create a nationwide stratum of public and private providers. Over 300 private primary care clinics have emerged and two thirds of the 30 commissioning agencies for the national insurance programmes, the *Entidades Promotoras de Salud* (EPS) are now private partnerships.

Much of the pump priming for this mixed economy, both ideologically and financially, has come from the likes of the Kellogg Foundation and the Inter-American Development and World Banks. In addition, universities such as that of Santiago de Cali have promoted forms of community governance so that health and social care professionals can come together with local citizens in approved State Social Enterprises that are an equivalent to semi-autonomous NHS trusts in the UK. These are an important source of social solidarity, sometimes supported by supplementary local insurance schemes, in a country that has been devastated by drugs wars with deaths from 'external causes' (usually violence) reaching 40 000 per annum.

Colombia is a classic example of the new political significance of health professionals' extended relationships. The collaborations required here at the northern tip of South America are, of course, particularly vivid given the local context, but they are not extreme: simply one end of the spectrum that applies everywhere to the resourcing imperative of modern health systems development. The universal pattern for these collaborative relationships is that of a *network*. As the likes of Microsoft and Virgin have demonstrated, network organisations can be highly successful. They can retain their corporacy and coherence while gaining hugely in flexibility over past models of bureaucratic and business organisation. They do this through unified information systems that support links between people which are often remote, transitory and tactical. Such networks can sustain an infinite number of collaborations. They are the cornerstone of integration.

Clinical and care networks now abound. Nowhere are they more evident or necessary than in Greece, where every health professional likes to describe every other health professional as 'my very good friend'. It would be unwise not to. One regional director in Athens described to us the Greek health decision-making process as like 'pulling strings from behind the curtain'. In a country with less than 11 million people but over 60 000 doctors (the second highest in Europe, behind Spain which unlike Greece proactively exports its medical manpower), and every type of health and social care funding, collaboration is the name of the game and the means of profitable survival.

Every day, every week, every month, the network of the Greek health professional grows. Loosely coordinated at the level of 17 regional systems, the *Periferiaka Systimata Ygias*, where the core patient database systems are held, the post-April 2001 modernised National Health Service (EYS) has sought to harness the benefits of bringing together all forms of resource investment. Doctors can use most public hospitals for private treatments at a 40% surcharge every afternoon. Now 20 000 run their own fee-for-service clinics with automatic reimbursement eligibility to many of the 30 occupational and geographical insurance schemes operating across the country. Mixed status specialists including general medical practitioners combine in the 300 new polyclinic style service network centres operated by the Ministry of Social Affairs (IKA). Some of the staff here also belong to the local authorities' community health teams which bring together social workers, home carers and community nurses, using European Union pilot funding. And then there are the hospital 'feeder' outreach clinics sponsored by charities, the medical centres and the provincial hospitals covered by national taxation, and the public-private partnerships of the target 400 Diagnostic and Treatment Centres. For every health professional there is a veritable portfolio of simultaneous career opportunities across the contemporary services network.

To the outsider, as the Greek experience amply illustrates, this emerging network of health professionals can be almost indecipherable. To understand how it operates often requires an appreciation of the informal relationships in Greece. Over half of the population are graduates, so these relationships are often rooted in the local university's curricula and what are termed 'circles of influence'. The lack of apparent visibility and clarity should not be confused with a lack of performance. Greek health status compares well with virtually every other country's. Likewise, Colombia's reform process is arguably the most progressive of the Latin American countries. Networks today are the most sophisticated source for the collaborations required of health professionals with a whole range of new partners. They enable the relationships with these partners to be integrated through the impartial sharing of information across disciplines and the opportunistic exploration and exploitation of non-formal as well as official contracts. As with equity, therefore, integration has the global scope to become an ethical as well as an economic motif of the future professionalism in health and social care.

With policy actors

The resource dividends of new professional networks with different partners require the support and stimulus of policies for integration that can contribute effectively to collaboration through the organisational arrangements they create. Globally these arrangements are increasingly being conceived of as *systems*. The relationship between inputs and outputs (or outcomes) needs to be understood by taking into account the complexity of variables of the throughput processes, their interactions and the interplay with impinging forces from the external environment. We have seen above how the term *sistemata* has been applied to the provincial level of health management in Greece. In Zambia, Ghana, Kenya and many other African countries both medically and nursing trained Clinical Officers coordinate the work of service outlets run by local government, NGOs and local communities in District Health Systems, while in such developed countries as Denmark, Israel, Sweden and England 'whole systems thinking' has become the basis for comprehensive and long-term health improvement programmes.

In the same way that integration takes health professionals into new collaborations with new agencies so the systems approach introduces them to whole sectors such as education, media and communications; as well as the voluntary sector. The 'Towards Unity for Health' WHO supported global movement looks to capture this new relationship diagrammatically in its 'Partnership Pentangle'. Shown in Figure 3.1, this sets out very simply the way in which the inter-sectoral relationships of modern health systems need to be conceptualised, and then operationalised as a network.

This 'Pentangle' offers a collective framework for health professions to belong to the 'virtual' or 'learning organisations' through which contemporary health systems are developed. They themselves become policy actors, planning together in cross-boundary teams for future contingencies, modelling alternative scenarios,

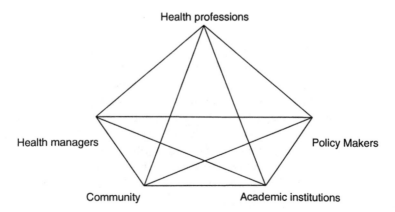

Figure 3.1 Partnership Pentangle.

and taking advantage of unexpected opportunities. Health professions of all kinds are far more involved in strategy, management and leadership than ever before. This is often now through such interprofessional associations as the NHS Alliance in England or genuinely multi-sectoral coalitions like the Maastricht based Network of Community Partnerships for Health through Innovative Education, Service and Research. WONCA, predictably, foresees the future general practitioners enjoying a pivotal role as coordinators and leaders within what Department for International Development (DFID) has coined the 'Sector-Wide Approach' (SWAP)[7]. Its advocates argue as follows:

> 'One of the main challenges faced by those working to improve health systems is the reconciliation of divergent viewpoints and entrenched interests among a variety of partners. Government health authorities, health service managers, health professionals, academic faculty members and community representatives each provide indispensable contributions for the development of a coherent, responsive and sustainable health system. To build productive relationships among these partners, strategies are needed to address differences in perspectives and to resolve conflicts that often result in fragmented, dysfunctional health systems.'
>
> (Boelan *et al.*, 2002, p. 3)

One such 'fragmented, dysfunctional health system' has been that of the Philippines where 'WONCA style' general practice has never taken root. Here in what, paradoxically, is the country with the highest global rankings for both religious observance and violent crime, health is indivisible from other public service issues. The only way in which health professionals can enhance the efficacy of their own services, with health expenditure at less than 3.5% of GDP in 2002, is through participation in cross-sectoral policy forums and development programmes. Security, welfare, hygiene, basic education and, above all, poverty are the issues.

Accordingly, under the terms of the post-1991 Republic of the Philippines Code of Decentralisation, District Physicians-in-Charge at local health centres are responsible for occupational health and environmental health alongside food safety, sanitation and the full range of primary medical care services. They and their professional colleagues serve on the local governing boards (LHBs) of the Code's 1700 defined geographical units for public service management, alongside NGO, community and ministerial representatives and elected local councillors for health. At national level, too, they join with private pharmaceutical, not-for-profit HMO and Government personnel to agree the Philhealth quality assurance criteria that should (but often do not) apply to the accreditation of any service outlet, whatever its status. And finally, on top of these critical collaborative roles in operational and regulatory policy, Filipino professionals fully participate

---

[7] SWAP has become the mantra for UK Government aid to such countries as Zambia, Kyrgyzstan and Uganda. It allows the external donor to intervene to ensure that both individual professional and economic developments are subject to honest and effective public administration, which ties health care advances to sustainable anti-poverty (and corruption) development strategies. See Fransen (2001) and Jeppson (2002) for specific country examples of this approach.

alongside international donors, aid organisations, universities, other Government departments and traditional mission based societies on the independent Council for Health and Development at Quezon City. This promotes, trains and helps coordinate a nationwide network of health service referral and information points, which again each have their own cross-sectoral local committees and 'Friends Groups'. Termed Community-Based Health Developments (CBHDs) these collaborations involve, via a National Field Support Unit, Medical School volunteers from as far away as Norway and Belgium, through to administrative emergency planning and relief support from the Japanese national Government.

In the Philippines the *learning organisation* and the *Sector-Wide Approach* come together in what convening health professionals call 'round table discussions'. Anybody can attend and contribute, no matter what their origin or affiliation: the table is circular so that there are no sides. Across it, at different angles and different levels, everybody can make contact and any subject can be put onto the surface of the table.

The results are tangible and easily visible. In Manila there are dedicated shopping malls of health and social care facilities which stretch from health insurance and facilities companies to physician clinics and community pharmacies (e.g. Ortega's Medical Plaza). Out on the islands the multi-purpose Barangay Health Workers draw on every sort of public/private/voluntary supplier for their stores of vitamins, contraceptives, vaccines and drugs (including for example, Rotary International, USAID and Pfizer). Cross-sectoral collaboration is almost without limits in a country which is regarded as a global leader in its modernising approach to health systems decentralisation.

With public representatives

Pragmatically, cross-sectoral collaboration, as exemplified by the Philippines, where it is a no-alternative requirement, offers governments more management and monetary resources for their health and social care professionals to draw upon. Presentationally, however, the pragmatic argument is not always attractive. Indeed there are many potential professional beneficiaries who object to the origins of some of the new offers of assistance. Both governments and professions regard themselves as publicly accountable, sometimes separately and sometimes through each other, but always fundamentally. All other forms of collaboration, except that with the individual citizen or patient, are of secondary significance. But equally, the unavoidable growth in the other forms of collaboration does compel a reframing of the public relationship.

The principle of *quality* is the vehicle for this reframing. Originally borrowed from the private commercial sector it is now embedded in the practice of modern health and social care professionals. As a marketing term for both themselves, and for governments, it has enabled the different and often competitive regimes of *managed care* to be introduced in ways that have offered the modern notion of *enrichment* to the public relationship.

Where this did not happen, in Russia, Portugal, Sri Lanka, Poland and parts of the USA, for example, managed care is associated in the public mind with reduced service and investment levels. The impact of new technologies and scientific research is regarded as threatening not enriching. The absence of overarching quality approaches at governmental level has left professionals exposed to new consumerist (and communist) reactions in their most negative forms[8].

Ignoring new technologies and evidence-based research is not an option for the modern health and social care professional. Neither is disregarding the modern quality principle and its conceptual supports. For example, the idea of enrichment ensures that the 'illness script' is multidimensional, not simply confined to technical interventions or physical symptoms. Enrichment enables clinical expertise to be augmented and encapsulated in frameworks which also include an understanding of prevailing (pre-) conditions; possible reasons for breakdown, and alternative outcomes. Such approaches respond to public perceptions of quality in health and social care, across the world, as being more about interpersonal values and attributes than technocratic factors[9]. Where such approaches have become successfully institutionalised in collaborative relationships between public representatives and health and social care professionals the results can be unexpected, encouraging and remarkably productive.

The WHO, accordingly, characterises health systems with this pattern of relationships as 'third generation': a maturation from market models enabling primary managed care methods to be legitimised even for such major public health threats as AIDS and malaria[10]. Finland is one of the few classic 'third generation' countries that have so far emerged. Its area health centres integrate the services of health and social care professionals. In most of the country's main population centres their management is combined. This is the land of Nokia and information systems, which allowed general practitioners to utilise computerised prescribing protocols and referral guidelines for nine out of ten of their cases more than a decade ago; the country where 'even health economists do not disagree' as consensus service strategies are developed through meticulous 'academic detailing' over three to five years. This is the 'family' nation where policy is progressed by public representatives and health and social care professionals in 'rainbow coalitions'[11].

---

[8] For a valuable overview of the impact elsewhere of USA based managed care models see Mechanic (2002) and Peterson and Swartz (2002). For individual country experiences refer, for example, to Twigg (2002), Jayasinghe *et al.* (1998) and Cabiedes and Guillen (2001).

[9] One excellent example of this, which also cites some of the international evidence, comes from the unlikely location of Guinea. See Haddad *et al.* (1998). For more detailed analysis of how models of enrichment lead, for example, to qualitative improvements in diagnosis and assessment see Feltorich and Barrows (1984) and Schmidt (2002).

[10] See WHO Annual Report (1999), Barnard (2002) and Peterson and Swartz (2002).

[11] The quotations given here come from our interviews with Finnish health professionals and policy makers in February 2002 at the Ministry of Health, Helsinki, Kangasala Health Centre, National Social Security Institute (KELA), and the Universities of Tampere and Helsinki.

In Finland quality is the thematic of health and social care, yet central surveil-
lance and monitoring by national Government is minimal. In their place are
profound and modern public-professional collaborations at the level of the muni-
cipality and the metaphor. Together these give a common shared meaning to the
system. Formally, health and social care is the responsibility of 440 municipalities.
The latter, for example, decide on the new professional appointments to a health
centre. But the relationship is a mutually dependent one. The health centre is
accredited by the local university health care faculty. The municipal councillors
and the medical school academics are partner custodians of the public interest
and this commonality is rooted in the quest for best quality. Together they invest
in the independent but quasi-governmental and world leading national Research
and Development Institute in Helsinki (STAKES – combining a health and social
care remit). They 'push each other's buttons' in a joint determination to obtain and
apply up to date information and guidance. Quality in Finland is 'the fairytale
that will never come true'; but in which the professionals, the politicians and the
public must nevertheless always believe, and for which they should forever
search.

Such idealist aspirations have a hard edge. Finland, comparatively, is a well
resourced country in terms of its health and social care, but it still has shortages of
frontline professionals in some of its more remote northern regions and resistance
to new working practices amongst general practitioners in its southern towns.
Private cooperatives, Swedish expertise and new nurse practitioner models have
had to be selectively imported to fill the gaps. In short, difficult decisions on
priorities and the limitations of a public service have had to be made. If this has
been necessary in Finland, then it is clear that no country is immune from the
rationing issues and mixed economy developments which can only be legitimised
by the public and their approved representatives. To remain at the forefront of
these modern health and social care developments, professionals must collaborate
and demonstrate their quality credentials.

With the patient

The building block for this collaboration at public levels, and indeed for each of
the other partnerships defined in this chapter, continues to be with the individual
patient. Globally this relationship, and the values that underpin it, are changing.
Historically the relationship has been associated with the linear model of diagnosis, treatment and cure. It has been characterised by hierarchical status, whether
this be, for example, in the mode of the super-specialist of Germany, the paternalistic general medical practitioner of the UK or the salaried state Soviet surgeons
suspiciously seen in the past as agents of social compliance and control. These
models and this status are now both unsustainable. Illness is a negotiation in
terms of its meaning and the responses required. Ownership remains with the
individual. The contemporary health and social care professional is in a change

agent role, to which collaborative relationships are critical if *trust* is to be achieved and nurtured.

This trust is multifaceted. Its modern expression reflects what the WHO policy makers describe and prescribe as the proper 'deconcentration' of power. This egalitarian concept goes far beyond simply signifying different forms of organisational decentralisation. Its twin is the notion of 'civil society'. In this framework of ideas, health and health care as individual rights are achieved through a personal and holistic sense of well-being in which medicine and formal professional providers are only one set of participants. Indeed, for this well-being, enhanced and expanded democratic forums of participation are pivotal. In these the patient is citizen first and foremost, with the forums ranging from single issue focus groups to local service management committees – all coming together to create what has been termed the 'sense of place'[11] wherein individual encounters with health and social care professionals are based on the maximum feelings of trust accumulated through: 'the perceptions, attachments and expectations individuals hold with respect to the local, or physical surroundings within which a particular activity or event occurs.' (Hanlon, 2001, p. 155)

The trust and collaboration with patients, as a result, is derived not simply from the practitioner's clinical focus and expertise. Communication channels, quality standards, levels of cooperation and even explicit patient oriented policies are also now equally important ingredients. In the Netherlands this modern concept of trust has been critical to the preservation of, for example, small general practice service units and through the medical faculties of such universities as Utrecht and Maastricht the Dutch have had a considerable influence on European thinking[12]. Throughout many parts of South America the collapse of political structures has frequently meant that civil society is being resurrected through a new richness in relationships with professionals, in the absence of public trust in government.

Peru is the leading example of this trend. It has over 2000 health centres, each managed by seven citizen Comités Locales de Administración de Salud (CLAS), which, by 2004, controlled (and helped to generate) more than a third of the country's health care expenditure. Six of the seven citizens are local patients; the other is the lead local professional (usually a public health doctor). The former are elected by the local community and by the Health Ministry (MINSA). Individually they assume lead roles for priority health problems and partnerships. Their collective decision-making powers stretch from prescription charges to professional appointments. They have been remarkably successful in expanding levels of both preventive and curative medicine, supporting community developments and contributing to a national civil society movement (Foro-Salud) which embraces large-scale regional and national citizens' health conferences, university faculties, municipal authorities and NGO sponsored

---

[11] (Hanlon, 2001) This term is often now used by advocates of more relational healthcare, e.g. The Cambridge Relationships Foundation.

[12] See for example Straton, Friele *et al.* (2002). Dutch University Institutes (e.g. NIVEL) have historically been the major recipients of EU Research Framework grant funds (particularly in primary care) and influential on policy developments as a result.

strategic planning[13]. In Peru this dispersal of influence represents a systematic deconcentration of power. It is an achievement still out of reach for such countries as Australia and Canada, where provincial state management structures operate as barriers; or indeed for NHS primary care trusts in England, where studies have found that lay representation at executive level is usually still a token single member, despite 'patient participation' being rated in 2002 as the most pressing priority for these new forms of what the Peruvians call 'social managerialism'.

Lessons

Having travelled the world in this chapter, let us come closer to home in addressing the overall lessons emerging from global policy developments in professional collaboration. In the UK, Prime Minister Tony Blair heralded his plans for a New National Health Service with a statement that characteristically combined practical and moral considerations: 'Our approach [to modernising the NHS] combines efficiency and quality with a belief in *fairness* and partnership.'(our emphasis) The Prime Minister in his Foreword to his Government's first major policy directive to those in the health professions went on to define this approach as the 'big challenge' in 'creating an NHS that is truly a beacon to the world' (Secretary of State, 1997, pp. 2–3)

It would be a dangerous mistake for health and social care professionals to equate such statements with political spin. Partnership and the collaborations that ensue are at the essence of future practice and development. As Tony Blair's words indicate this is both hard-headed pragmatism and heartfelt conviction because, as our global scan has sought to show, modern principles of policy and their supporting ideas are as robust and irreversible as those they succeed in moving from institution and market led health and social care environments to models of partnership.

Accordingly, professional *autonomy* now has to be earned and as a principle it acquires legitimacy through the response of those practising in health and social care to the collaborative challenges of *complexity* and *participation*. Similarly, *equity* as a relational principle means professions must not duck away from the issues of *substitution* and *distributional justice*. And so on through to the most important principle of all for professions: *trust*. A trusted health and social care professional is the patient's (information) guide. He or she recognises the new extent of his civil responsibilities as political power everywhere is deconcentrated in different processes of decentralisation and local resource management. In relation to trust, Peru is not just another interesting case example. It is the classic expression of

---

[13] For example, the US based NGO Future Generations has offices in Lima where its Directors Dr Ricardo Diaz and Dr Laura Altobelli assist CLAS development with regular evaluation and scenario planning. For a recent critical review see Iwami and Petchey (2001).

global forces and trends which require professionals to collaborate in their personal and local response.

Of course such global developments as have been considered in these chapters will be differently expressed in different contexts. Valuing diversity is a significant factor in contemporary collaboration and global policy drivers and determinants will vary in their impacts from individual continent and country levels right down to those of individual carers and clinicians. For the public health specialist, for example, the modern *systemic* principle may be most significant with its critical supporting ideas of *enrichment* and the *sector-wide* approach. For most nurses, by contrast, *quality* has been the motivational trigger, while for the cardiovascular surgeon, literally at the cutting edge of technological change, the capacity to integrate *transdisciplinary* knowledge across new professional *networks* may well be of most importance. In each and every instance the case for collaboration is now clear cut and global.

Conclusions

This chapter has sought to extend awareness and understanding of global forces and trends for collaboration. It has pointed to the growing significance of the WHO and associated intercontinental policy forums in promoting new forms of partnership. (Chapter eight provides readers with a more detailed account of these developments.) Through the triangular framework of six legitimising principles for modern health and social care and their pairs of key supporting ideas the themes of modernisation set out in Chapter one have been revisited through their expression in international initiatives. Individual country case examples have indicated both the breadth of the changes in collaborative practice for professions, and the potential for innovations. They have also pointed to some of the pitfalls and possible risks; the most serious of which is one that every health and social care practitioner will have witnessed in their professional practice: *denial.*

Bibliography

Barnard, K. (2002) *Public Health and the Challenge of Implementing Primary Health Care.* World Health Organization Report EUR/02/5037844/BD2, Geneva.

Boelen, C., Haq, C., Hunt, V., Rivo, M. & Shahady, E. (2002) *Improving Health Systems: the contributions of Family Medicine.* World Organisation of National Colleges and Academies, Geneva.

Bossert, T. (1998) Analysing the decentralisation of health systems in developing countries: decision space, innovation and performance, *Social Science and Medicine,* **47** (10), 1513–27.

Buchan, J. & Dal Paz, M. (2002) Skill mix in the health care workforce: reviewing the evidence. *World Health Organization Bulletin,* **80** (7), 575–580.

Cabiedes, L. & Guilten, A. (2001) Adopting and adapting managed competition: health care reform in Southern Europe. *Social Science and Medicine*, **52**, 1205–17.

Department of Health (1999) *National Service Framework for Mental Health: Modern Standards and Service Models for Mental Health*. Department of Health, London.

Exworthy, M. & Halford, S. (1999) Professionals and managers in a changing public sector: conflict, compromise and collaboration? In: *Professionals and the New Managerialism in the Public Sector*. (eds. M. Exworthy & S. Halford). Open University Press, Buckingham.

Feltovich, P. & Barrows, H. (1984) Issues of generality in medical problem solving. In: *Tutorials in Problem-Based Learing: A New Direction in Teaching the Health Professions* (eds H. Schmidt & M. De Valder). Van Goraum, Assen, The Netherlands.

Fransen, L. (2001) Partners in health and poverty. *Development*, **44** (1), 129–31.

Griffiths, F. & Sweeney, K. (eds) (2001) *Complexity and General Practice*. Radcliffe Medical Press, Oxford.

Haddad, S., Fournier, P., Machovf. N. & Yatara, F. (1998) What does quality mean to lay people? Community perceptions of primary health care services in Guinea. *Social Science and Medicine*, **47** (3) 381–94.

Hanlon, N. (2001) Sense of place. Organisational context and the strategic management of publicly funded hospitals. *Health Policy*, **58**, 151–73.

Harrison, S. & Pollitt, C.J. (1994) *Controlling Health Professionals*. Open University Press, Buckingham.

Health Service Circular (1999/123) *Governance in the New NHS: Controls Assurance Statement 1999/2000: Risk Management and Organisational Controls*. Department of Health, Wetherby.

Hobus (1995).

Iwami, M. & Petchey, R. (2002). A CLAS act? Community-based organisations, health service decentralisation and primary care development in Peru. *Journal of Public Health Medicine*, **24** (4), 246–51.

Jayasinghe, K., DeSilva, D., Mendis, N. & Lie, R. (1998) Ethics of resource allocation in developing countries: the case of Sri Lanka. *Social Science and Medicine*, **47**, 1619–25.

Jeppson, A. (2002) SWAP dynamics in a decentralised context: experiences from Uganda. *Social Science and Medicine*, **55** (20), 2053–60.

Kahssay, H. & Oakley, P. (eds) (1999) *Community Involvement in Health Development: a Review of the Concept and Practice*. World Health Organization, Geneva.

Meads, G. (1999) Streaming into the River. Network-based Development. *Journal of Inter-professional Care*, **13** (3), 271–6.

Lassey, M., Lassey, W. & Jinks, M. (1997) *Health Care Systems around the World: Characteristics, Issues and Reforms*. Prentice Hall, New Jersey.

Mechanic, D. (2002) Socio-cultural implications of changing organisational technologies in the provision of care. *Social Science and Medicine*, **54**, 459–67.

NHS Executive (1999) *Clinical Governance. Quality in the New NHS*. Department of Health, London.

Pan American Health Organisation (2002) Profile of the Health Service System of Columbia. WHO/PAHO Division of Health Systems and Services Development, Washington, DC.

Peterson, I. & Swartz, L. (2002). Primary health care in the era of HIV/AIDS. Some implications for health systems reform. *Social Science and Medicine*, **55**, 1005–13.

Schieber, G. & Maeda, A. (1999) Health care financing and delivery in developing countries. *Health Affairs*, **18** (3), 193–205.

Schmidt, H. (2002) *The Development of Expertise in the Health Sciences, Abstract*. 'The Network' Annual Conference, Moi University, Eldoret.

Secretary of State for Health (1997) *The New NHS. Modern, Dependable.* Department of Health, Cm 3807, London.

Straton, G., Friele, R. & Groenewegen, P. (2002) Public trust in Dutch health care. *Social Science and Medicine*, **55**, 227–34.

Twigg, J. (2002) Health care reform in Russia: a survey of head doctors and insurance administrators. *Social Science and Medicine*, **55**, 2253–65.

Walsh, W.B. (1998) Building public/private collaboration in China. *Health Affairs*, **17** (6), 6.

WHO African Regional Committee (1988) Document AFR/RC37/RI. Bamako Initiative, Mali.

WHO (1998) *Primary health care in the twenty-first century. Everybody's Business.* Report of Alma Ata Declaration 20th Anniversary Meeting, 27–8 November. Almaky, Kazakhstan.

WHO (1999) *Health Systems and Service Development.* World Health Organization Annual Reports, Geneva.

WHO Regional Office for Europe (2000) *Report on a meeting with WHO Collaborating Centres and Selected Organisations,* (September, Barcelona). World Health Organization, Copenhagen.

WHO/WONCA (2001) *Towards Unity for Health and Family Medicine.* Working paper based on the proceedings of the WONCA–WHO Collaboration Meeting in Durban, South Africa. May 17–19, p. 4.

World Bank (1993) *Investing in Health.* World Bank Report, Geneva.

Further Reading

Blas, E. & Limbambla, M. (2001) The challenge of hospitals in health sector reform: the case of Zambia. *Health Policy and Planning*, **16** (supplement 2), 29–43.

Boelen, C. (2000) *Towards Unity for Health: Challenges and Opportunities for Partnership in Health Development.* World Health Organization Report EIP/OSD/2000.9, Geneva.

Brommels, M. (2001) *Effective Professional Practice Behaviour: the Ultimate Managerial Challenge.* University of Helsinki, Helsinki.

Goicoehea, J. (ed.) (1996) *Primary Health Care Reforms.* World Health Organization, Copenhagen.

Johnson, D. (2001) *South Africa.* Department for International Development Health Systems Resource Centre Briefing Paper, London.

McIntyre, D. & Gibson, L. (2002) Putting equity in health back onto the social policy agenda: experiences from South Africa. *Social Science and Medicine*, **54**, 1637–56.

Mays, N. (2002) Reform and counter reform: how sustainable is New Zealand's latest health system restructuring? *Journal of Health Services Research and Policy*, **7** (supplement 1), 46–55.

Morgan, L. (2001) Community participation in health: perpetual allure, persistent challenge. *Health Policy and Planning*, **16** (3), 221–30.

Secretary of State for Health (1997) *The New NHS. Modern, Dependable.* Department of Health, Cm 3807, London.

UNI-SOL (1999) *Weaving Global Links.* Health Sciences Center, University of Arizona.

Widdus, R. (2001) *Public-Private Partnerships for Health: Their Main Targets, Their Diversity and Their Future Directions.* World Health Organization Bulletin, **79** (8), 713–20.

Section II
Practice into Policy

In this section we explore in depth the management agenda for collaboration by and between health and social care professionals, drawing upon specific recent examples from national public inquiries and performance reports, and illustrative international case studies.

Rosalind Scott, John Ashcroft and Andrea Wild

4 Crisis Prevention

Purpose

Failures of collaboration can occur because professionals are too busy and under pressure. Hastily written up notes can be incomplete, an important conversation or telephone call can easily be forgotten in the midst of a busy day. Such failures are routine: collaboration can break down at any point in any team. The risks are compounded by weaknesses in systems and culture. It is not simply a few incompetent individuals who fail to collaborate, it could be anyone in any country.

Sometimes the consequences are severe: patients can die; careers are blighted; organisations are named and shamed. The purpose of this chapter is to demonstrate for health and social care professionals how easily failures of collaboration arise; to explore the consequences of these failures and to understand how collaborative failures can be avoided.

Professionals may be held accountable for their own collaborative failures, as well as for failing to ensure effective collaboration by others. The Kennedy Report into the high mortality of children undergoing paediatric cardiac surgery (PCS) at Bristol found that:

> '...relations between the various professional groups were on occasions poor. All the professionals involved in the PCS service were responsible for this shortcoming. But, in particular, this poor teamwork demonstrates a clear lack of effective clinical leadership. Those in positions of clinical leadership must bear responsibility for this failure and the undoubtedly adverse effect it had on the adequacy of the PCS service.'
>
> Kennedy (2001) Summary point 24

Collaboration is essential in every area of health and social care to avert tragedies such as those reviewed in this chapter. Any analysis of collaboration must consider the direct factors which affect interpersonal collaboration and the other factors which determine the structures and systems that enable effective collaboration. These include, for example, record keeping to support good interpersonal communication and systems which encourage collaborative working practices. As explained in Chapter two (pp. 18–31), collaboration needs to be strategic, not merely structural.

Theoretical models for analysing adverse events

There is a growing body of research about how to analyse adverse events and the importance of reporting and learning from 'near misses,' that is incidents which almost happened.[1] This research stresses the need to analyse the reasons for adverse events in terms of failures of systems and chains of events rather than as isolated incidents conducted by incompetent individuals. After 1997 the UK Government set up a Patient Safety Agency to this end and in 2004 combined its functions with the National Institute for Clinical Excellence (NICE) working alongside the Commission for Social Care Inspection (CSCI) and the Commission for Healthcare Audit and Inspection (CHAI). All of these bodies seek to improve the quality of clinical treatment and ensure its regulation. The trend to ensure safety has resulted in the development of a series of models which are commonly used to analyse adverse events. These models, which are reflected in the Inquiries' analyses, highlight a range of factors, some of which directly relate to the inter-personal relationships between parties. Others such as organisational and systems factors relate to the context for effective collaboration. As with the research about adverse events itself, the models tend to prefer a complex whole systems approach which identifies both contributory general factors, such as organisational context, and specific failures.

This is apparent, for example, in the 'Swiss cheese model of organisational accidents' developed by Reason (1990, 1997, 2000). The model is based on the premise that while all the barriers to ensure safety should be intact, they are actually patchy like Swiss cheese and contain holes. When the 'holes' (in the cheese) in each system line up, they allow a brief 'window of accident opportunity' during which dangerous situations can arise. It is acknowledged that, in healthcare especially, there are often very few barriers to accidents: for instance when a nurse administers a drug to a patient. The model identifies both human factors, for example, miscalculating the dosage of a drug, and pre-existing organisational factors such as the dispersed location of clinicians who work together. There are, therefore, 'latent conditions' which can align themselves and create conditions whereby an 'active failure' by an individual is more likely.

Vincent *et al.* (1998, 2000a) built upon Reason's model to demonstrate that it is the interaction of a variety of factors which tends to result in an adverse medical incident. He identified a series of categories of factors: institutional context which includes the economic and regulatory frameworks of the NHS in the UK, organisational and management factors, work environment, team factors including written and verbal communication, supervision and team structure, individual (staff) and task factors. In addition Vincent developed a protocol for care management problems which are actions or omissions by staff during the care process. This categorisation can be used to classify clinical context and patient factors, specific contributory factors and general contributory factors.

---

[1] See example (Department of Health, 2000)

Alternative means of analysing adverse events have been developed by Helmreich and Higgins, amongst others. Helmreich (2000) identified four types of poor conduct which increase risk: poor communication, poor leadership, conflict in interpersonal relations and poor preparation, planning and vigilance. Higgins (2001) identified certain patterns of failure which recur when adverse events are analysed: isolation, poor leadership, lack of exposure to new ideas, systems and processes (failure to observe procedures), poor communication and disempowerment (Walshe & Higgins 2002). These are relational themes and their link to failures of collaboration is explored in more detail below. Isolation precludes collaboration. Poor leadership will be seen in the failure of clinical leaders to work as part of their teams and in failing to ensure that other collaborate effectively. The lack of exposure to new ideas and best practice is symptomatic of limited and parochial collaboration that excludes the contribution of those who can enable improvement. We will describe repeated failures of systems and processes to sustain effective collaboration in complex situations. We will give examples of poor communication that resulted in failure of inter-agency collaboration and see how the disempowerment of individuals or professions prevented concerns from being raised effectively.

Sources and methodology

The main focus of this chapter is to examine the events leading up to the death of Victoria Climbié and the failure by the United Bristol Hospital Trust (UBHT) to save more infants suffering from congenital heart disease. The main sources are the public inquiry conducted by Lord Laming into the death of Victoria Climbié and that of the public inquiry conducted by Professor Kennedy into the death of children in Bristol[2]. This chapter draws on these reports to identify the lessons for collaborative practice elsewhere. It does not, and should not, examine again the roles and responsibilities of any of the local individuals involved in either case.

These two contrasting examples have been chosen because they address the breadth of provision within health and social care. Victoria Climbié received hospital treatment and was referred to Social Services. The Bristol Inquiry considers aspects of the work of Bristol Royal Infirmary, an acute service, in more detail. The inquiries have been influential in leading to new service arrangements (such as Children's Trusts which bring together services across health, education and social services), more integrated regulation and inspection, as well as advocating significant workforce reforms.

There are, of course, many other inquiries that could have been considered. There is a whole literature of mental health inquiries into the harming of patients themselves and others by patients suffering from mental illness[3]. In addition, a

---

[2] See evidence submitted to the Public Inquiry into the death of Victoria Climbié, Final Report, 2003 and the Final Report of the Bristol Royal Infirmary Inquiry by Professor Kennedy, 2001.

[3] For a full list of all inquiries into the death of mentally ill patients since 1985 see www.davesheppard. co.uk. A selection are referenced in the Bibliography at the end of the chapter.

comprehensive international literature exists which documents adverse events such as the Presidential Inquiry undertaken in America. This inquiry found that at least 44 000 and perhaps as many as 98 000 people die in hospital each year as a result of preventable medical errors (Kohn *et al.*, 2000). A great deal of research has also been undertaken in the United States into the importance of teamwork[4]. In Europe, a series of academics have been working on the need for collaboration[5]. In addition, many administrative and computer failures in the UK and abroad have led to a whole series of errors related to screening, including non detection of women with abnormal cells during breast- and cervical screening procedures. The focus of this chapter will be British public inquiries. There is insufficient space here to consider the international literature, although extensive examples of healthcare systems in other countries are discussed in other chapters of the book.

THE INQUIRIES

The Bristol Royal Infirmary Inquiry

The Public Inquiry by Professor Kennedy found that a series of flaws surrounding open-heart surgery carried out on children at Bristol Royal Infirmary 'led to around one third of all the children who underwent this surgery receiving less than adequate care.' In the period from 1991 to 1995 'between 30 and 35 more children under 1 died after open-heart surgery in the Bristol Unit than might be expected had the Unit been typical of other PCS units in England at the time.' Figure 4.1 shows the network of care for neonatal patients suffering from heart disease and the external bodies responsible for monitoring performance.

The Inquiry identified shortcomings in both the surgery and intensive care, failures to identify and address these shortcomings within the hospital trust, as well as shortcomings in the external monitoring of the quality of care. The relationship with parents was also criticised with regard to giving consent, provision of support and counselling, and the way in which concerns about treatment were handled. Whilst strongly criticising some individuals, the Kennedy report emphasised their good faith and the influence of systemic failings. The report's synopsis describes the combination of factors that contributed to these failings.

> 'The story of the paediatric cardiac surgery (PCS) service in Bristol is not an account of bad people. Nor is it an account of people who did not care, nor of people who wilfully harmed patients. It is an account of people who cared greatly about human suffering, and were dedicated and well-motivated. Sadly, some lacked insight and their behaviour was flawed. Many failed to communicate with each other, and to work together effectively for the interests of their patients. There was a lack of leadership, and of teamwork. It is an

---

[4] See for example Heinemann & Zeiss (2002) who have developed 50 instruments to measure (inter-professional) team performance.
[5] See for example work by Engeström & Ovretveit (1997).

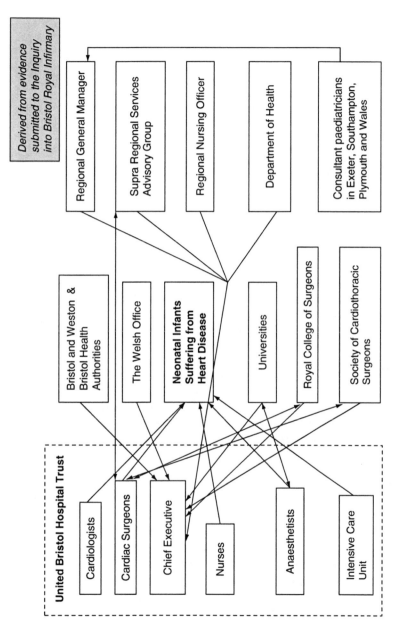

Figure 4.1 The network of care for neonatal patients suffering from heart disease.

Table 4.1   Selected timetable of events: Bristol.

1984	Bristol Unit designated as a supra-regional service for neonatal cardiac surgery
1986	South Glamorgan Health Authority raise concerns about quality and reluctance to refer
1987	Exeter's reluctance to refer notified to region
1989	Anaesthetist raises concerns and starts to collect data
1992	Series of articles referring to PCS in Bristol published in Private Eye
1994	Letter signed by six anaesthetists expressing concern about arterial switch programme at BRI
1995	Advisability of proceeding with operation on a junior male patient discussed. Operation goes ahead and patient dies. Surgery suspended. Extensive media coverage of the story. Helpline established
1998	Secretary of State requests Inquiry

account of healthcare professionals working in Bristol who were victims of a combination of circumstances which owed as much to general failings in the NHS at the time than any individual failing. Despite their manifest good intentions and long hours of dedicated work, there were failures on occasion in the care provided to very sick children. It is an account of a service offering paediatric open-heart surgery which was split between two sites, and had no dedicated paediatric intensive care beds, no full-time paediatric cardiac surgeon and too few paediatrically trained nurses. It is an account of a time when there was no agreed means of assessing the quality of care. There were no standards for evaluating performance. There was confusion throughout the NHS as to who was responsible for monitoring the quality of care. It is an account of a hospital where there was a 'club culture'; an imbalance of power, with too much control in the hands of a few individuals. It is an account in which vulnerable children were not a priority, either in Bristol or throughout the NHS. And it is an account of a system of hospital care which was poorly organised. It was beset with uncertainty as to how to get things done, such that when concerns were raised, it took years for them to be taken seriously.'

Kennedy (2001) Synopsis paras. 3–10

The long lead-in time for failures of collaboration is indicated in Table 4.1 by the Bristol time line. This illustrates how the various factors identified by Vincent can come together effectively, and calamitously. Task factors can be seen in the inherent risks in paediatric cardiac surgery. Individual factors included the clinical leadership of the cardiac surgeon. Team factors were seen in the lack of multidisciplinary teams and the lack of openness which made it difficult for junior doctors to raise and discuss concerns. The work environment was influenced by the split site and limited resources. Organisational and management factors were reflected in the 'silo' structure and club culture which hindered a multiprofessional approach to reviewing quality of care. The wider institutional context included the lack of an effective system for external monitoring of quality and what Klein has described as 'an NHS culture that encouraged heroic endeavour against the odds and the acceptance of inadequate resources as the norm.'

This, Klein argued, resulted in the ethos of 'getting by', the dedication of health professionals to do their best, even with inadequate buildings, staffing and equipment, becoming the enemy of excellence.[6]

The Victoria Climbié Inquiry

Victoria Climbié came to England with her great aunt, who was her guardian and pretended to be her mother. In April 1999 she was seven and a half years old. Victoria had significant contact with no less than six public services comprising two hospitals, three local authorities and the police. Others, such as health visitors, should have had contact with Victoria but the referral was neither logged nor acted upon. Figure 4.2 displays the relational network of care for Victoria Climbié and the complexity of the relationships. The Counsel for the Inquiry identified 12 missed opportunities by public services to save Victoria. In the words of the Laming report 'the dreadful reality was that these services knew little or nothing more about Victoria at the end of the process than they did when she was first referred to Ealing Social Services by the Homeless Person's Unit in April 1999' (Laming, 2003:3).

Victoria spent much of the last weeks of her life wrapped in a bin liner, lying in a bath with her faeces and urine, with her hands and legs tied. She was regularly beaten, with the post mortem recording 128 separate physical injuries. The failure to conclusively detect abuse and protect Victoria by many agencies over a period of ten months resulted in Victoria's death on 25 February 2000. Both Victoria's aunt and her aunt's partner were subsequently convicted of murder.

Laming (2003:40) concluded that 'the extent of the failure to protect Victoria was lamentable. Tragically, it required nothing more than basic good practice being put into operation. This never happened.' While Laming found that 'the standard of work done by those with direct contact with [Victoria] was generally of very poor quality' the strongest criticism is reserved for 'the managers and senior members of the authorities whose task it was to ensure that services for children, like Victoria, were properly financed, staffed and able to deliver good quality support to children and families.'

This, then, is a story of failures of effective interprofessional and inter-agency collaboration in the context, for some of the organisations, of 'deep-rooted deficiencies' which meant that staff were working 'in an under-resourced, under-staffed, under-managed and dysfunctional environment' (Laming, 2003:85) Emphasising the importance of collaboration Laming concluded that:

'The future lies with those managers who can demonstrate the capacity to work effectively across organisational boundaries. Such boundaries will always exist. Those who are able to operate flexibly need encouragement, in contrast to those who persist in working in isolation and making decisions alone. Such people must either change or be replaced.

---

[6] 'No Quick Fix', *Health Service Journal* 30 August 2001 p. 29.

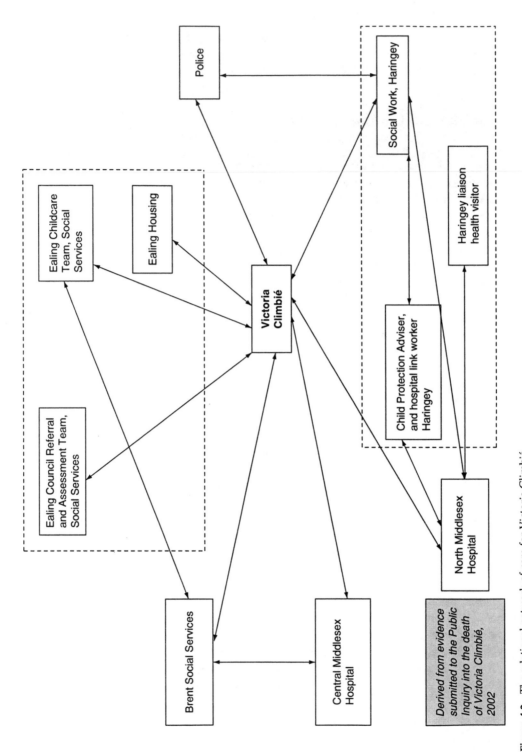

Figure 4.2 The relational network of care for Victoria Climbié.

The safeguarding of children must not be placed in jeopardy by individual preference. The joint training of staff and the sharing of budgets are likely to ensure an equality of desire and effort to make them work effectively.'

Laming (2003:8)

Laming sought 'to secure strong local working relationships so that collaboration on the scale of that which I envisage takes place' by proposing mechanisms to ensure that clear ability for outcomes drove collaboration. These led to the introduction of new legislation and the establishment of local Children's Trusts. The vision for these pathfinders is described as:

'Multi-disciplinary teams based in universal services such as clusters of schools or early years settings... A shift to prevention while strengthening protection...Practical changes underpinned by clearer accountability and partnership. By a cultural transformation to create more trusting relationships between frontline professionals – doctors, nurses, teachers police and social workers...This places duties on every agency to work together to deliver common outcomes.'

Department for Education and Skills (2004) *Every Child Matters: Next Steps* p. 3

In order to make sense of the lessons for the key interprofessional relationships that are the focus of this book it will be helpful to summarise some of the key aspects of Victoria's story, and the interactions between professionals and agencies that occurred.

Victoria and her aunt attended the Ealing Homeless Person's Unit on 1 May 1999 where a narrow assessment for emergency housing assistance was made. She was placed in temporary housing in Brent. The first anonymous call to Brent Social Services indicating concern about Victoria's welfare was made on 17 June 1999. Signs of a child in need[6] were detected but the referral was delayed for three weeks and seriously mishandled. There were no written records to prove that enquiries had been made of Ealing Social Services and Housing Departments, a GP or other health professionals. The lack of information meant that the social worker who visited Victoria's home on 14 July 1999 had no details about the referral or information about the possible indicators of abuse. Victoria and her aunt had moved into her aunt's new partner's bedsit a week earlier so Victoria was not seen.

Victoria was, in fact, taken to the Central Middlesex Hospital on the day of the abortive visit by the daughter of her childminder. A medical report on a child 'thought to have suffered abuse' and a body map of injuries was faxed to Brent Social Services. No link was made to the previous referral but Victoria was placed under police protection, albeit without a full assessment being made. A consultant paediatrician then diagnosed scabies. The notes were written by a registrar who wrote *no child protection issues* when what was meant was *no physical abuse issues*. The notes were not checked by the consultant. The inquiry found no evidence to

---

[6] Signs of a child in need include bed wetting, physical injury, non school attendance and poor living conditions. These signs were detected by Ealing and Brent Councils but not acted upon.

dispute the diagnosis of scabies but concluded that signs of physical abuse should also have been detected. The difference of wording proved significant. The medical diagnosis and assessment of abuse was not questioned by social services, and police protection was withdrawn without a full investigation.

After Victoria was discharged from Central Middlesex Hospital, her case was not transferred back to Ealing Council in order that a Child in Need assessment be carried out. There are no written records to indicate that this transfer took place. At the time no machinery existed to ensure the systematic exchange of information about children in need across boroughs. The authorised procedures were not followed which resulted in the loss of important information about child protection concerns that arose during admission to the Central Middlesex Hospital. Victoria was discharged into the care of her aunt. The inquiry found that 'the result of this obviously inadequate approach to Victoria's discharge was that she left hospital without any record of her departure, without a discharge letter, without having been seen by a social worker, and without any arrangements whatsoever being made for any form of medical or nursing follow-up' (Laming, 2003:253).

Within days of discharge from the Central Middlesex Hospital, Victoria was admitted to the North Middlesex Hospital on 24 July 1999. Victoria was admitted for two weeks but a full investigation was not conducted during her stay, nor was the full nature of the medical staff's concerns and suspicions made clear in writing to social services. A joint police and social services check on the safety of discharging Victoria to her home was not made. Many concerns by both doctors and nurses were not fully recorded in Victoria's notes, hindering the ability of other staff to pick up on concerns and allowing misapprehensions to continue. Laming concluded that:

> 'The management of Victoria's care at the Central Middlesex Hospital and the North Middlesex Hospital was full of inadequate and ambiguous recording of information and actions, deferred actions, assumptions and expectations that things 'would happen' or be done by 'someone' or others 'at a later stage'. There were numerous failures to ensure that things they thought would happen did happen. Victoria's case clearly demonstrates the need for doctors and nurses to document information, actions and referrals consistently and unambiguously, to share that information, and to ensure subsequently that what has been agreed is carried through.'

> Laming (2003:283)

Victoria's case was not picked up by either the GP or health visitors due to the inadequate referral. Two visits were made by a social worker who was not aware of the seriousness of child abuse concerns and incorrectly believed that the earlier scabies diagnosis (from Central Middlesex) addressed the concerns raised by North Middlesex. The last attempt to correct this misunderstanding was made on 2 November 1999. This was the last involvement any health professional had in Victoria's case until she returned to North Middlesex Hospital on 24 February 2000, the evening before she died.

Framework: key sets of relationships

The public inquiries can usefully be analysed using the six collaborative relationships for professionals outlined in Figure 4.3. These are the professional relationship with same profession, with other professions, with (new) partners, with policy actors, with the public and with patients. Before proceeding, it is important to draw a distinction between a relationship with another profession and a relationship with a (new) partner. The former is essentially contingent upon achieving a specific goal. For example a hospital consultant will write to a GP about a particular episode in a patient's medical history. The relationship ends when the patient is discharged. It is patient specific. By contrast, a relationship with a (new) partner indicates a relationship which *pre-exists* the presence of any individual patient or client. It is inter-organisational, for example the police and social services have an ongoing relationship in order to investigate child protection cases. Most relationships among partners also entail an interprofessional dimension but this is not the sum of the relationship.

With same profession

The two inquiries raise a number of important lessons for collaborative relationships with members of the same profession. These include the support provided to more junior staff, the dangers of 'silo' structures that impede horizontal communication and the way in which concerns about performance should be raised. Whilst such factors as split sites, inadequate resourcing of services and management systems are cited by the inquiries as significant factors, the need for cultural change was also singled out. Effective teamwork, focused around the needs of the patient and reinforced by clear and appropriate accountability, was seen as essential in ensuring that legitimate expectations about quality of care are met.

Consultants and junior doctors must work together effectively to provide quality of care. Shortcomings in these relationships were noted in both inquiries. There were no dedicated intensive care beds for children at Bristol Royal Infirmary and the particular collaborative requirements for care for very young babies

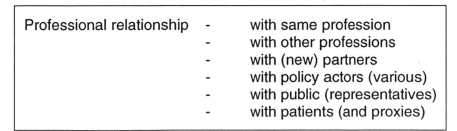

Figure 4.3   Key sets of relationships.

were not met. The junior doctors who were physically present in the Intensive Care Unit for most of the time did not have ready access to experienced colleagues to address the more rapidly changing condition of babies (Kennedy, 2001:215). There were also cultural problems in the relationship at Bristol with the Inquiry finding that there was a mindset among younger clinicians that 'older established consultants had been left behind by recent developments', with a 'degree of resentment and defensiveness among the older consultants if practices were challenged' and that the 'club culture' created an 'environment that was not such as to make speaking out or openness safe or acceptable' (Kennedy, 2001: 165). This is echoed in the Inquiry finding that 'exhaustion and low morale lead to stagnation and an inability to move forward in response to new developments [in other PCS services], despite the stimulus provided by the new generation of consultants' (Kennedy, 2001:231).

Split site working also affected the care of Victoria Climbié with the consultant covering two units. When staff work shifts in hospitals it may be very difficult to find an opportunity to have a face to face discussion about a patient. Advice, sharing of information, and follow through of decisions can suffer as a result. When there are staff shortages a consultant may be on duty at one hospital while technically on call at another. This meant that 'a locum junior hospital doctor, with little knowledge of local child protection procedures, was left unsupported at the Central Middlesex Hospital and allowed to handle alone Victoria's discharge from hospital.' The Laming report (2003: 1.57) goes on to describe this as 'totally unacceptable. No member of staff, from any of the agencies, should be put in a position that places both them and their client, or patient, in such a vulnerable position.' Patients now need to be discharged at the explicit consent of a consultant, following the recommendations, but this was not the case when Victoria Climbié was admitted to the Central and North Middlesex Hospitals.

Effective collaboration requires time and good communication. Although the children at Bristol were admitted under the joint care of cardiologists and surgeons the 'meetings between cardiologist and surgeon were a casualty of the cardiologists being overstretched.'[7] The consultant paediatric cardiologist reported that being based on different sites limited 'the ordinary communication that exists in a unit where consultants and various doctors can meet with each other and bump into each other in a corridor, and so on, which facilitates the overall management' (Kennedy, 2001:212). Advice from cardiologists at critical moments during surgery was not readily accessible.

The Kennedy report (2001:231) also found that 'there was poor understanding of the importance of teamwork, most particularly in the case of collaboration between cardiologists, anaesthetists and surgeons in the management of ICU; that teams are necessarily multidisciplinary.' Shortfalls in teamwork were compounded by 'the uneasy relationship between anaesthetists and surgeons.' The difficulties the anaesthetist encountered in raising his concerns were described by the Inquiry as revealing 'both the territorial loyalties and boundaries within the

---

[7] There was a significant national shortage of paediatric cardiologists at the time.

culture of medicine and of the NHS, and also the realities of power and influence' (Kennedy, 2001:161).

Improving performance requires that a broad view is taken of the care provided and that the whole system is analysed as well as the constituent parts. At Bristol, if there had been more insight into the collaborative endeavour which the cardiac surgeon and his colleagues were engaged in, he may well have been able to investigate the poor performance more objectively and may have been less defensive about the PCS outcomes. Strict vertical hierarchies within clinical directorates can mean that junior colleagues are unable to question or even validate consultant assessments. At Bristol the cardiac surgeon appears to have genuinely believed that it was the complex medical conditions which patients presented rather than the overall quality of care which resulted in poor PCS outcomes. This analysis from the leadership, coupled with his leadership style, seems to have prevented open discussion of clinical standards, hindering the development of corporate strategies to improve clinical outcomes. 'The net effect of these various arrangements was that they clearly militated against the development of a strong body of information and analysis that would have enabled healthcare professionals to look across the boundaries of the various specialities to assess the care provided by multi-disciplinary teams' (Kennedy, 2001:235).

Another instance of interprofessional collaboration requiring conscientious communication is highlighted by the Consultant's diagnosis of scabies at the Central Middlesex hospital. In a busy hospital where different professionals work different shifts there is often little time to discuss changes which are made to diagnosis. In the case of Victoria Climbié, however, this diagnosis was extremely important and inadvertently led to the dropping of two child protection investigations. The Consultant did not discuss the diagnosis with colleagues who had indicated possible non-accidental injuries. Lack of face-to-face interaction and shortcomings in the medical notes across all the medical staff involved in Victoria's care meant that a clear and agreed account of actual or suspected abuse was not made. Lord Laming's recommendations state that in such situations any misunderstandings about diagnosis should now be corrected in writing.

With other professions

Collaboration is also required across disciplines and professions. Weaknesses in the relationship between medical professionals subsequently hindered the relationship with professionals in other agencies. The need for all interested parties to share information and for written communication to clarify all verbal communication of significance is essential in preventing ambiguity and misunderstandings. The Climbié Inquiry found that there was a manifest lack of 'a clear understanding by all parties involved as to exactly what information needs to be communicated and within what timescale...' Protocols can be developed which assist professionals to share information. These include clear instructions about who to contact within an organisation, for example a social worker or hospital linkworker. The two inquiries demonstrate that clarity about the role and responsibility of each professional working on a case, including identification of overlaps requiring particular collaboration and early identification of any gaps in the service provided, is of paramount importance.

In the case of Bristol there was a sharp distinction between clinical and managerial responsibilities as well as a 'silo structure' that impeded horizontal communication. The chief executive who instituted this structure was a strong believer in clinical freedom and autonomy.

> 'Leadership in Bristol was fragmented; clinical leaders were expected to take responsibility for discrete areas of clinical care; managers were expected to focus on non-clinical matters. A separation was created which was hard to sustain. Delegation of authority from the Chief Executive to clinical directorates created 'silos' (discrete organisational units with very little communication between them) within the Trust. These were almost separate organisations. Strategic leadership from the centre was weak. Communication was up and down the system but not across it.'
>
> Kennedy (2001:302)

Collaboration between professions is one of the key control factors against risk. At Bristol, however, nursing staff 'were let down by a culture that excluded them.' The Kennedy report (2001: 175) concluded that 'the hierarchical system common at the time (and regrettably still too prevalent now) made it difficult for the nursing staff to voice concerns and to be heard.' That nurses would refuse to scrub for some operations but have no other adequate means of pursuing their concerns is testimony to the lack of a multi-professional approach to ensuring quality of care. The Inquiry found that the Director of Operations combined this role with that of Nurse Adviser to the detriment of the duties associated with the latter. The 'club culture' excluded nurses who had no effective advocate for their concerns (Kennedy, 2001:201).

'Teamwork is the collaborative effort of all those concerned with the care of the patient. Patients do not belong to any one professional; they are the responsibility of all who take care of them' (Kennedy, 2001:277). Chapter two noted the importance of having an appropriate focus for collaboration. At Bristol the patient was not the focus. Although 'the consultants, particularly the surgeons, saw themselves as having very effective teams' the inquiry found that they saw them as their teams, which they *led* but were not *part of*, other than as leaders. The inquiry also found that the teams were 'teams of like professionals: consultant surgeon leading surgeons, consultant anaesthetist leading anaesthetists. The teams were not organised primarily around the care of the patient, they were not cross-speciality nor multidisciplinary, and they were profoundly hierarchical' (Kennedy, 2001:198).

As Chapter two indicated, poor communication can arise because of a lack of parity between different professionals which makes open exchanges difficult. In the case of Victoria Climbié, the effects of the scabies diagnosis were underestimated. The combination of the lack of clear written communication of suspected emotional (and possible physical) abuse and the hierarchical relationship between different professionals meant that suspicions were not acted on. Both the social workers from Brent and Haringey felt unable to question the medical diagnosis of a Senior Consultant. It is reasonable to assume that they would have been more alert to the danger facing Victoria if they had been provided with a fuller briefing. In response to this the Laming Inquiry recommended that 'the training of social workers must equip them with the confidence to question the opinion of professionals in other agencies when conducting their own assessment of the needs of the child.'

This example highlights the importance of interprofessional parity and the difficulty of fostering this when relationships are brief and contingent. The discharge summary diagnosing scabies was faxed; the social workers received the information and allowed it to influence their investigation. There was, however, no significant interaction (at most a hurried telephone call) between the professionals, which made establishing priority very problematic. By contrast, the Linkworker from Haringey Social Services did meet the Consultant Paediatrician at the North Middlesex Hospital fairly frequently at meetings so the relationship preceded the particular events relating to Victoria Climbié. The Consultant brought Victoria's case to the Linkworker's attention in person, which provided the opportunity for an interaction about the particular case. The Linkworker in this instance *did* feel able to raise the discrepancy between the diagnosis of non accidental injury from the Consultant at the North Middlesex Hospital and the earlier diagnosis of scabies from the Consultant at the Central Middlesex Hospital.

To return to Reason's Swiss cheese model for a moment, it can be demonstrated that if a failure of collaboration occurs, for example the non-recording of information or a misdiagnosis, a hole appears in the cheese. Good collaboration can compensate for poor collaboration. If, for example, a clear diagnosis of non-accidental injury and been provided by North Middlesex Hospital, the hole opened by the first diagnosis of scabies could have been closed. Instead, the diagnosis of scabies was followed by unclear verbal communication and delayed letters to the Linkworker which did not reach the Social Worker; these factors combined led to the dropping of child protection concerns. The window of accident opportunity which appears to have opened up when the holes in the Swiss cheese lined up, was that child protection concerns could be set aside in spite of the existence of physical abuse due to a lack of clear and unambiguous communication.

With (new) partners

The case of Victoria Climbié illustrates the difficulties that can arise when many agencies are involved. Although the link between hospital and social services is not new, the systems were weak and compromised by failings in internal communication and processes, and the individual conduct of the relationship was at times poor. No-one was clearly and consistently responsible for protecting Victoria and in possession of the full range of critical information that had been gleaned piecemeal by different individuals and agencies. In responding to the 'gross failure of the system' with regard to the death of Victoria Climbié, Lord

Laming (2003: 1.42) made proposals 'designed to ensure that those who manage services for children and families are held personally accountable for the effectiveness of these services, and for the arrangements that are put in place to ensure that all children are offered the best protection possible.'

It became evident in the Inquiry that there was some uncertainty about who had lead responsibility. The relationship between the police and one Social Services Department was reported to be strained at times. The presumption that strategy meetings should always be held at social services offices was an illustration of a 'subservient approach' that 'seriously compromised [the police] ability to carry out robust, speedy and effective criminal investigations' (Laming, 2003:313). The nature of the relationship with social services was one factor in the 'entirely inappropriate' abandoning of a serious investigation 'because of a third-hand medical report [the scabies diagnosis] told to the [police constable] over the telephone' (Laming, 2003:302). Evidence to the Inquiry was regarded as demonstrating 'very clearly the dangers to children if staff from different agencies do not fulfil their separate and distinctive responsibilities. No set of responsibilities is subordinate to one another, and each must be carried out efficiently and effectively. Gathering together staff in a dedicated team requires that they all fully recognise and respect each others' responsibilities' (Laming, 2003:6).

Laming (2003:306) expressed concern 'that the good intentions of multi-agency decision-making, information sharing and joint working may now have lead to a blurring of roles, uncertainty about who should take what action, and a convenient excuse for poor investigation.' As we have seen in Chapter two, collaboration can legitimise and enable specialisation. Thus, Laming concluded, it was wrong for police to rely uncritically on medical staff to gather information necessary for criminal investigation (which was the police's specialist expertise), and for social services staff to allow a medical diagnosis to replace their own responsibility for ensuring a full Child in Need assessment.

In the light of Vincent's model for analysing adverse events (Vincent et al., 1998, 2000a) we should see collaborative relationships between partner agencies that are multi-layered. The task needs to be seen in terms of the whole needs of the person, as opposed to being defined by the contribution of the single profession or agency. Individuals must see their role as contributing to these outcomes, and having the skills and experience to do so. There will, at times, be the need for teams that cross agency and professional boundaries. There is a managerial responsibility to ensure work environments that can sustain the collaborative endeavour, and to ensure that appropriate systems are in place, resourced and monitored. This will be aided by a policy, regulatory and cultural environment that supports joint working. There were failings at all of these levels in the case of the collaborative relationships between partners which contextualised the care of Victoria Climbié.

Shortcomings in communication and the allocation of tasks and responsibilities illustrate the problems. The duty Senior Worker from Haringey Council attended the first Strategy Meeting in July 1999 because Victoria's file had not yet been allocated to a specific social worker. The Police Constable requested a full medical report after seeing the North Middlesex Hospital diagram of Victoria's body. The Police Constable assumed that a hospital social worker would ensure that the medical report was produced and circulated. The July Strategy Meeting was not held in the hospital and none of the hospital staff were able to be present, including the Consultant. Police participation was not, Laming found, at a sufficiently senior level to ensure the agency played its full and proper role. The tasks were not appropriately allocated and no-one was appointed at the meeting to check that all tasks had been completed in order to avoid confusion. The record of both the Strategy Meetings was not rapidly circulated. This did not then generate a case conference where the consultant paediatricians would have been required to attend. If the case conference had taken place in November or December involving social services, police and health professionals Victoria's care needs might have attracted different responses.

Paediatric cardiac services in Bristol involved fewer relationships with partners, in part reflecting the rather more limited relationships with primary care and commissioning authorities than that which developed throughout the NHS in subsequent years. Recognising that a period in hospital is only one element along a continuum of care, the Inquiry noted the weakness of the partner relationships at the time. 'We argue for the development of a more integrated approach to the provision of support services, whereby the respective roles of the hospital, the GP and local primary care team, the local Social Services Department and the various volunteer organisations are clarified and organised around the needs of the patient' (Kennedy, 2001:294).

The relationship between the two sites within the United Bristol Hospitals Trusts (the Bristol Royal Infirmary where the surgery was carried out and the Bristol Royal Hospital for Sick Children where the paediatric cardiologist was based) nevertheless has many of the characteristics, and problems, of deepening integration between new partners. The Inquiry found 'that the dislocation of essential cardiological services from the surgical and other services at Bristol Royal Infirmary was, in our view, one of the most significant adverse factors affecting the adequacy of PCS services overall.' PCS services were provided within the constraints of this relationship for over ten years despite acknowledgement of the difficulties and dangers that it posed. Where the nature of a relationship between partners unavoidably creates difficulties for service provision there is the danger that through both becoming accustomed to the problem and conditioned to working with these constraints, the commitment may diminish to either ensuring their effective resolution or questioning whether the partnership is in fact the best context for the provision of that service.

With policy actors

Chapter five looks in more detail at the importance of collaboration for maintaining and monitoring performance. It is important to consider the failure to monitor performance at Bristol Royal Infirmary here as well because this failure allowed the problem to persist, and more children to die during or after treatment, than if the poor performance had been detected and addressed. A series of organisational, management and institutional factors contributed to the persistence of the problem.

The Bristol Inquiry acknowledged that 'the prevailing wisdom was that policy-makers and managers should keep out of matters involving professional judgement. One such matter was the quality of service delivered. That was the preserve of professionals' (Kennedy, 2001:74). The anaesthetist at Bristol who was struggling to get his concerns about PCS addressed wrote to the Department of Health, but the letter was not read as this was seen as a local matter in which the Department should not be involved. There was confusion about the distinctive roles and responsibilities of each of the players and, in the course of the Inquiry, the NHS Executive accepted some responsibility for not clarifying them. The Inquiry's assessment of the state of the relationship with and between policy actors is blunt:

> '[No] organisation took responsibility for what a layperson would describe as keeping an eye on things. The SRSAG thought that the health authorities or the Royal College of Surgeons were doing it; the Royal College of Surgeons thought that the SRSAG or the trust were doing it, and so it went on. No one was doing it. We cannot say that the external system for assuring and monitoring the quality of care was inadequate. There was, in truth, no such system.'
>
> Kennedy (2001:192)

The Supra Regional Service Advisory Group (SRSAG) was responsible for overseeing the development of services and fulfilment of designation criteria in all hospitals providing supra regional services. SRSAG policy was to improve the quality of outcomes by increasing the volume of operations, which was not reviewed in spite of ongoing poor performance. This policy failed to take account of the other factors which, apart from surgical expertise, could affect performance such as the split site.

Confusion arose from SRSAG's data collection and the introduction of annual service agreements. They appeared to be involved in a comparative audit of services but they did not have the facility to monitor quality and act upon the information that they obtained. The Bristol Inquiry also found that the SRSAG did not effectively address or act upon widespread concerns raised by Consultant Paediatricians in Exeter, Plymouth, Southampton and Wales about referring patients to Bristol for treatment. The policy to increase the volume of PCS outcomes was never reconciled with this reluctance to refer patients to Bristol. The consultants and the SRSAG acted independently of one another. A failure of collaboration between professionals and policy makers contributed to the mismatch between policy and practice.

'The principal failure to protect [Victoria Climbié] was the result of widespread organisational malaise.'[8] Laming (2003:4) found that elected councillors and senior managers in the local authorities involved 'allowed the services for children and families to become seriously under-funded, and they did not properly

---

[8] Coming 2003:4.

consider the impact this would have upon their front-line services.' He did not accept the view that because 80% of their funding came from local government, and because they were being pressed to address central government priorities, that they had little scope to influence spending at a local level.

Nevertheless, the relationship with the centre, and the lack of collective accountability for outcomes for children either locally or centrally was an issue. The police acknowledged in the course of the Climbié Inquiry that monitoring of child protection teams was patchy and that until child protection was added to the Home Secretary's Police Priorities List, attention was likely to be focused on centrally determined targets. The introduction of the new childcare legislation is intended to mark a new role for Government in promoting change. 'For too long we have focused on micro-managing localities through small budgets and planning regimes. Our role in making change happen must be primarily as a catalyst and enabler' (Department for Education and Skills (2004) *Every Child Matters; Next Steps* p. 4).

This is seen in terms of:

- Sharpening the incentives and accountability for improving outcomes
- Rationalising targets to ensure all services are judged on how they cohere to meet common objectives through a new integrated inspection system
- Freeing up local practitioners through streamlined performance management, rationalised funding streams, new powers to pool budgets and share information, and tackling bureaucratic burdens
- Promoting change through actively sharing learning and investing in the workforce.

In promoting effective collaboration the relationship with policy actors should serve other relationships, most importantly the requirements of the relationship between services and public and patients. Laming summarises the challenge of putting the relationship with the public centre stage:

> 'Local government in this country should be at the forefront of organisations serving the public. Sadly, little I heard persuades me that this is so. Many of the procedures that I heard about seemed to me to be self-serving – supporting the needs of the organisation, rather than the public they are set up to serve. Local authorities should take the lead in promoting social regeneration and combating social exclusion. In this regard, I have recommended that local authorities become more closely engaged with their local communities in defining local needs and the ways to meet them. Little I heard in this Inquiry convinced me that local authorities accept that in public service, the needs of the public must come first. This must change.'
>
> Laming (2003:11)

With the patient

We have already noted that at Bristol collaborative working was not focused around the needs of the patient, however much individual medical staff may have been dedicated and hardworking in the care of their patients. A key factor in the failure to protect Victoria Climbié was that no agency had a robust continuous relationship with her and adequately assessed her needs. The relationship with her was at times subsumed under the relationship between services and her aunt, who was masquerading as her mother. Poor collaboration can weaken the relationship with the patient, but this relationship should also be seen in collaborative terms. The state of this relationship can be a symptom of breakdown, but also has the potential to protect against it – particularly when empowered patients can identify and negotiate the cracks in the system. Many service failures occur in the care of those who are most vulnerable, and consequently often least able to fulfil this role. We have seen in Section one of this book that the 'Modernisation' of services is changing the basis of the relationship with the patient under the banner of such themes as choice and accessibility of services. The Bristol Inquiry considered the information given to patients (in this case their parents) and the approach to gaining consent and recommended that a greater degree of partnership in the relationship should be established. 'It can no longer be acceptable for patients, having been treated, as they are now for the most part, as equal partners by their GP, then to go into hospital and be confronted with old-style paternalistic attitudes from some consultants' (Kennedy, 2001:285). The Royal College of Nursing and the Royal College of Surgeons argued in the course of the Inquiry that the development of skills to enhance partnerships with patients was vital.

This is not always easy, not least, as the Inquiry acknowledged, because patients cannot be expected to follow some standard model. One may want detailed information and explanation of risks. Another may not. There is also the practical problem of time. 'There is a relationship between the time to communicate and the resources available to the NHS. Time is a resource like any other resource. In the context of an NHS which has endured decades of constrained resources, the allocation of time to communicate with patients, though readily recognised by healthcare professionals as important, has been consistently squeezed' (Kennedy, 2001:290).

Time pressure is perhaps more easily managed when the patient is physically present, commanding attention. But the relationship with the patient is not simply a series of personal encounters (whatever the quality of those encounters) but also a continuous relationship with one or more agencies. It is a relationship that needs to be sustained by effective systems and communication. It is too easy for the relationship with a patient to become reduced to 'the random passing of slips of paper' (Coming, 2003:9). In seeking more systematic care Laming concluded that:

'The accurate and efficient recording of information cannot be left solely to the individual diligence of the doctors and nurses concerned. They must be supported by a clear system that minimises the risk of mistakes and provides a mechanism for recognising mistakes when they occur. The greater pressures are on staff, the greater the need for a system to support them. The busier the organisation, the more important it is to have a system that ensures agreed actions are recorded and completed.'

Laming (2003:283)

Another danger for this relationship is that patients (or their proxies) can be dishonest and manipulative. The Climbié Inquiry found that Victoria was sometimes only spoken to in the presence of her aunt and appeared to have been coached in her answers. The social worker from Haringey admitted to being misled by the aunt, particularly after the aunt informed her about the scabies diagnosis which was confirmed by the Central Middlesex Hospital. Victoria's aunt and her partner worked very hard to present themselves as a stable and caring family unit and to some extent they succeeded in this.

The final lesson for this relationship is dealing with the relationship when it goes wrong. There is concern that a more litigious culture precludes open and honest discussion of actual or possible mistakes with those who are affected by them. The risk is that an important feedback learning loop is lost, and greater costs incurred when issues are not resolved at an early stage. Partnership is all too easily lost when things go wrong. The conclusion of the Bristol Inquiry was to distinguish 'a system in which all interaction with patients becomes routed through a complaints system, such that comments become complaints, even if they did not begin as such, and a system which allows multiple opportunities for communication between the hospital and those it serves' (Kennedy, 2001:298). The future was seen to lie in the latter.

Lessons

Many of the failures of collaboration which have been identified above can be avoided. Professional vigilance on the part of individuals and the development of systems which enhance collaboration are necessary to avoid the failures and tragedies described in this chapter. Standardised forms make record keeping quicker and more accurate. Good record keeping means recording observations, telephone calls and face-to-face conversations. Poor record keeping is a significant failure of communication which can trigger a whole series of other errors. Centrally held records are a necessity and can contribute to a holistic and seamless service.

A management structure which fosters interdisciplinary working practices is essential to promote interprofessional collaboration. For specific services it is, however, necessary to separate clinically expert roles from those with responsibility for regulation in order to ensure impartial performance reviews. The management of all organisations should develop a constructive approach to audit as a means of measuring performance on an interprofessional basis. Protocols should be designed which encourage interpersonal information sharing. Reading records and following instructions are basic forms of collaboration which are fundamental, yet often overlooked by hard pressed professionals. Where possible it is important to nurture a culture of interprofessional parity characterised by greater face-to-face contact between professionals. The explicit allocation of tasks avoids confusion and designating a person with responsibility for ensuring the completion of all tasks reduces error. Managers ought to monitor outcomes and have the flexibility to review policy if there is no improvement. The purpose of all data collection should be clear and the supply of data for audit should be regarded as normative. Procedures should be in place at every level to investigate and improve poor performance.

Conclusion

As we have seen in this chapter, collaboration is essential in providing continuity of care. Failures of collaboration occur, not simply because individuals are incompetent, but because they are too busy and because they do not prioritise communication. Often a failure of collaboration appears to be a small oversight, such as not making notes of a conversation or not discussing a change of diagnosis, but as we have seen the consequences can be far reaching and tragic. Responsible health and social care professionals need to be both proactive in setting up systems and identifying weaknesses in advance, and to react rapidly to prevent a crisis when collaboration breaks down.

The shift of mindset is away from an individualised, self centred and task focus towards a willingness to work for the development of the team or the common good. This requires a generosity of spirit and an appreciation of the dividends of collaboration. Where collaborative working practices and systems exist, mistakes can be quickly corrected and a crisis averted. Collaboration can reduce error and lead to the introduction of a system of checks and balances among professionals which minimise risk. Collaboration cannot be left in the interpersonal domain. It must be inculcated in systems which promote interprofessional working practices. Professionals are often stretched to the limit of their capacity and steps are being taken since 1997 to redress a shortfall in the supply of health professionals in the UK[9]. It is within this climate however, that the imperative of collaboration needs to be taken on board. Collaboration can be a matter or life or death. It is essential, not optional.

We now move on in Chapter five to examine the relationship between collaboration and performance management, expanding our examination of some of the issues arising from the case studies in this chapter. The second section of the book concludes with Chapter six which considers the development agenda within interprofessional learning and some of the specific educational initiatives that have taken place across international health systems to promote the advance of professional collaboration.

Bibliography

Bourns, I. (1997) How can we learn from medication incidents? *Health Care Risk Report*, **3**(1), 18–20.
Chapman, J. (1996) *System Failure*, Demos, London.

---

[9] See, for example, Department of Health (2001a), Department of Health (2003b).

Department for Education and Skills (2004) *Every Child Matters: Next Steps*. HMSO, London.

Department of Health (1998) *A First Class Service: Quality in the new NHS*, HMSO, London.

Department of Health (2000) *An Organisation with a Memory, Report of an expert group on learning from adverse events in the NHS chaired by the Chief Medical Officer*, HMSO, London.

Department of Health (2001a) *Building a safer NHS for patients*. HMSO, London.

Department of Health (2001b) *Learning from Bristol: the report of the Public Inquiry into children's heart surgery at the Bristol Royal Infirmary 1984–1995*. HMSO, London.

Department of Health (2003a) *Keeping Children Safe, the Government Response to the Lord Laming Inquiry*. HMSO, London.

Department of Health (2003b) *Every Child Matters*. HMSO, London.

Engeström, Y., Engeström, R. & Vähäaho, T. (1999) When the center does not hold: the importance of knotworking. In: *Activity, Theory and Social Practice*. (Ed. by S. Chaklin, M. Hedegaard & N.J. Jensen). Aarhus University Press, Aarhus.

Helmreich, R. (2000) On error management: lessons from aviation. *British Medical Journal*, **320**, 781–785.

Heinemann, G. & Zeiss, A. (2002) *Team Performance in Healthcare: Assessment and Development*. Kluever Academic, New York.

Higgins, J. (2001a) Adverse events or patterns of failure. *British Journal of Health Care Management*, **7**(4), 145–147.

Higgins, J. (2001b) The listening blank. *Health Service Journal*, **111**, 22–25.

Hornby, S. & Atkins, J. (2000) *Collaborative Care*. Blackwell, London.

Kennedy, I. (2001) *Final Report, Bristol Royal Infirmary Inquiry*, HMSO, London.

Klein, R. (2001) No Quick Fix. *The Health Service Journal*. 30 August 2001 p. 29.

Kohn, L., Corrigan, J. & Donaldson, M. (2000) *To Err is Human: Building a Safer Health System*, National Academy Press, Washington D.C.

Lord Laming (2003) *The Victoria Climbié Inquiry: Report of an Inquiry by Lord Laming*. HMSO, London.

Ovretveit, J., Mathias, P. & Thompson, T. (1997) *Interprofessional work for health and social care*. Macmillan, Basingstoke.

Lupton, C., North, N. & Khan, P. (2001) *Working together or pulling apart? The NHS and child protection networks*. Policy Press, Bristol.

Reason, J. (1990) *Human Error*. Cambridge University Press, Cambridge.

Reason, J. (1997) *Managing the risks of organisational accidents*. Ashgate, Aldershot.

Reason, J. (2000) Human error: models and management. *British Medical Journal*, **320**, 768–770.

Rosenbloom, M. (2003) Medical Error Reduction and PDAs. *International Paediatrics*, **18**, 2, 69–77.

Sexton, B.J., Thomas, E.J. & Helmreich, R.L. (2000) Error, stress and teamwork in medicine and aviation: cross sectional surveys. *British Medical Journal*, **320**, 745–749.

Sloan, S. J. (1997) An Occupational Psychology Perspective on Risk Management. *Health Care Risk Report*, **3** (4), 21–24.

Vincent, C. (2001) (Ed.) *Clinical risk management: enhancing patient safety*. BMJ Books, London.

Vincent, C., Neale, G. & Woloshynowych, M. (2001) Adverse events in British hospitals: preliminary retrospective record review. *British Medical Journal*, **322**, 517–519.

Vincent, C., Stanhope, N. & Taylor-Adams, S. (2000a) Developing a systematic method of analysing serious incidents in mental health. *Journal of Mental Health*, **9** (1), 89–103.

Vincent, C., Taylor-Adams, S., Chapman, E.J., Hewett, D., Prior, S., Strange, P. & Tizzard, A. (2000b) How to investigate and analyse clinical incidents: Clinical Risk Unit and Association of Litigation and Risk Management protocol. *British Medical Journal*, **320**, 777–781.

Vincent, C., Taylor-Adams, S. & Stanhope, N. (1998) Framework for analysing risk and safety in clinical medicine. *British Medical Journal*, **316**, 1154–1157.

Walshe, K. & Higgins, J. (2002) The use and impact of inquiries in the NHS. *British Medical Journal*, **325**, 895–900.

Wilson, J. (1996) Clinical Risk Management in General Practice. *Health Care Risk Report*, **3**(1), 19–21.

5 Performance

Introduction

Performance is the more positive ambition that balances the requirement to avoid service failure. The term can, however, provoke an ambivalent response. The language of performance can have a positive image: it is the language of achievement, fast cars or sporting success. But for some people, and many health and social care professionals in our experience, the dominant image of performance is of play-acting, removed from reality and working to someone else's script. In a similar vein targets may also be associated with negative images, tainted with the perception of intrusive reductionism and limited ability to capture the ethically driven commitment to care and serve.

Maintaining and improving performance can be seen simply as satisfactorily achieving objectives and meeting the legitimate expectations of those who have a stake in health and social care. This is important for both personal and organisational success, as well as for society as a whole. Underperformance is penalised, while high performance offers a range of rewards. For the health professions, job satisfaction, reputation, career progression and pay are at stake. For organisations, their future funding and development may rest on how their performance is assessed. For patients it may be understood in terms of the quality and accessibility of the care that they receive. And for elected representatives, politically accountable for the performance of the health system, it may dictate whether or not they remain in office. One common theme here is that performance builds confidence and trust. How one performs, or is perceived to perform, will shape the future pattern of key professional relationships.

The first part of this book has argued that policy now requires collaboration; which is shaping accounts of performance, although policy themes and approaches to assessing performance are not fully integrated. This chapter starts by looking at one local performance assessment framework to illustrate how pervasive the case for collaboration is becoming. What needs to be done cannot be done alone. Having considered what should count as performance we will then consider some of the factors that influence performance, with particular reference to the impact of collaboration. In the light of this we then consider the implications of the concern for performance for each of the six key relationships (with same profession, other professions, partners, policy actors, the public and patients), that are the chief focus of this book. Two main sources of material are used: the UK experience of changing performance management in health care and a wider international literature on performance in other sectors.

What counts as performance?

Understanding what drives, or should drive, the concern for performance helps health professions to respond in ways which support the collaborative relationships that are key to improving health. The five themes of modernising health systems outlined in Chapter one therefore set the context for this discussion of performance, as follows:

- Local resource management shifts the location of performance management with, for example, greater interest in whether local needs and priorities are being addressed
- Governance introduces new accountability structures, resulting in new approaches to monitoring and communicating performance
- Integration makes cross boundary partnerships both an objective to be assessed and the context within which other aspects of performance can be assessed
- Stewardship for public health creates one major set of performance goals or targets
- Quality focuses on both clinical care and access to care as key outcomes to be assessed

These themes are illustrated in the national planning priorities in England and Wales[1] and their local application. Table 5.1 sets out the main performance areas addressed in these planning priorities. Each area has a number of performance indicators, examples of which are shown to illustrate the implications for collaboration. Separate sets of performance indicators are produced for NHS primary care trusts, acute (hospital) and specialist trusts, mental health trusts, ambulance trusts, and social services (Commission for Health Improvement, 2002). Examples of the local implications for delivery are taken from Cambridge City NHS Primary Care Trust, chosen as the chapter author's local area (Cambridge City Primary Care Trust Local Delivery Plan, 2003–2006). While the details of the plan reflect the peculiarities of the UK context, it illustrates a wider principle that improvements in quality (the definition of which we will consider in more detail below) cannot be achieved in isolation.

---

[1] DoH (2002). In the UK, after a period when performance targets changed annually and often reached three figures, the national priorities are now set for a three-year period and total six to eight. Curiously this greater focus seems to have added to professional pressures and reduced individual freedoms.

Table 5.1   National Planning Priorities: implications for collaboration and local delivery.

National plan theme	Examples of collaboration required	Examples of collaboration in local delivery plan
Access	Collaboration between partners to improve choice and reduce waiting times	• Participate fully in the Emergency Care Collaborative • Work with our hospital trusts to ensure maximum A&E wait reduced to four hours
Cancer	Interprofessional and partner relationships in developing care pathways	• Enhance primary care lead support to ensure effective links within primary care and between primary and secondary care services • In conjunction with other localities agree additional consultant support and networking relationships within palliative care
CHD	More defibrillators commissioned in public places	• Review the initial phase of scheme to develop network of community first responders • Review provision of health promotion initiatives in schools and community settings
Mental health	Expanding capacity in provision of crisis resolution, assertive outreach and care for prisoners	• Continue joint working to reduce current rates of suicide in line with national suicide prevention strategy • In conjunction with social services and others review use of selected beds with a view to providing more appropriate care in the community
Older people	Working with partners to improve care at home and reduce hospital admissions	• Develop a more integrated approach to community health and social care that allows for flexibility to meet individual needs • In conjunction with social services and others purchase additional equipment to facilitate better care packages in the community/at home
Children	Ensure the NHS and local government work together to improve life chances for children	• Work with social services and other agencies to ensure that Quality Protects plan targets are achieved • Commissioning community development schemes in line with the project plans agreed with the national Sure Start unit
Patient experience	Strengthen accountability to local communities	• Satisfy ourselves that key providers are demonstrating quality improvements in their performance • Continue to work with city council to pursue opportunities for joint consultation using the city council's Citizen's Panel

(Continued)

Table 5.1   (*Continues*)

National plan theme	Examples of collaboration required	Examples of collaboration in local delivery plan
Health inequalities	Improved access for disadvantaged groups (through partnerships)	• Play a full role in the work of the Local Strategic Partnership and achieving its objectives • Work in partnership with child and family nurses to minimise the risk of social exclusion
Drugs	Working with partners to increase participation in drug treatment programmes	• Cross-cutting issues to be addressed are overdose, blood-borne viruses, psychiatric co-morbidity, outreach work, criminal justice systems, users, carers and self-help groups
Physical facilities	Introduce new providers from the independent sector and overseas to offer patients greater choice	• Offer greater choice by agreeing referral shifts and shifts of inpatient and day case workload • In conjunction with the city council and others agree plans to establish a Healthy Living Centre
Workforce	Increase workforce capacity and productivity through skill mix, professional development and substitution	• Pilot the integration of nursing teams across primary, community and social care services • Developing partnership with the Anglia Support Partnership; the knowledge management and library service to give staff access to best practice and best evidence information electronically
IM&T	Collaboration between health and social care agencies and suppliers to deliver new systems	• Prepare for the introduction of electronic prescriptions • Support the development of secure information exchange between health and social care partners
Value for money	Cost efficiency increases of at least 1% a year	• 'We are relying on the success of modernisation initiatives to help us improve the efficiency of services, do things differently and to yield the balance of the funding required either through savings or through avoiding the need to invest.'

Derived from Cambridge City Primary Care Trust Local Delivery Plan, 2003–2006.

The first point to note is that it is organisations and services that are the main focus of performance assessment. Greater public availability of data on individual consultants is proposed. This will include, for example, information on waiting times for outpatient appointments. The key national indicators illustrate the need for collaboration in that, for example, primary care trusts are assessed with respect to the number of outpatients waiting longer than the standard – something which can only be addressed together with the relevant acute and specialist trusts. The local response to this agenda requires many examples of collaboration. An overview of this is provided by the local PCT's ten 'strategic aims' (Cambridge City Primary Care Trust (2003) p. 6). Specific references to collaborative relationships include: 'We will have created a seamless approach to the provision of support for adults with chronic illnesses and older people by working in partnership with our colleagues in social services and the voluntary sector'; or: 'We will have a close collaborative relationship with Addenbrooke's, other NHS trusts and neighbouring PCTs to deliver better health care services to the local community'.

The details of the local delivery plan indicate that the other strategic aims also have significant collaborative requirements. As illustrated in Table 5.1 these include investing in partner agencies, integrating services, partnerships for health promotion and supporting the development of new interprofessional relationships and ways of working. Health outcomes require the contribution of all the six professional relationships that are the focus of this book. If improved health outcomes are the goal, the touchstone for performance, then the case for collaboration is inescapable. The concern for performance in health and other public services is not, however, always experienced as closely linked to outcomes. The process can divert time and distort activity. Organisational or service targets may be hard to reconcile with the needs of the individual to whom there is a strong ethical and professional commitment. The case for collaboration here is to shape the definition of performance as well as to satisfy its requirements. If different concerns and priorities cannot be integrated within the context of collaborative relationships then the experience of performance management will be, at least for some professions and organisations, an imposed agenda.

The importance of recognising diverse perspectives on quality was summarised in the London King's Fund report on quality in general practice. Perspectives discussed included those of the reflective practitioner, the patient, the 'activity' perspective, the 'gatekeeper', the prescriber, the educational perspective and the management perspective:

> 'The notion of a unitary, one-dimensional index that can be used for assessment of all aspects of quality is a dangerous illusion. Different interest groups increasingly concede that their different objectives necessarily require different measures of quality, and this paper is, first and foremost, a recognition of the plurality of perspectives that are already beginning to exist. Acknowledging the lack of universality of one's own paradigm, as well as understanding and respecting alternative perspectives on the issue, is a more important step towards constructive dialogue than any attempt to achieve a forced consensus.'

> (Greenhalgh and Eversley, 1999 p. 3)

The definition of performance and the processes for assessing it must capture the range of concerns and viewpoints. Failure to achieve this can easily lead to alienation, not least amongst professional groups. In many sectors there is a shift towards a more broad-based account of performance exemplified in, for example, balancing reporting on financial performance with indicators of corporate social responsibility. The balanced scorecard, used in both public and private sectors, offers one example of this, in providing a clear prescription as to what organisations should measure in order to 'balance' the financial perspective[2]. Typically this monitors performance from four perspectives, with one application tailored for public services, describing these as customer, capacity, process and financial (personal communication of author in 2003). The aim is not simply to map what has gone wrong, but rather to provide a diagnosis linked to outcomes that are rooted in mission and strategy. There are a number of factors which influence these different perspectives and the understandings of quality to which they give rise.

(1) **Accountability**

This influences who sets the purpose and thus the overall direction of the account of performance. The challenge for health professions is to deal with different accountabilities and their potentially conflicting accounts of performance. The interests of an individual patient will not always be easy to reconcile with community-oriented public health priorities or the requirements of a health care organisation with its own set of accountabilities.

(2) **Purpose**

Any account of performance must be rooted in the overall goals of that organisation or service. This statement of purpose (mission) may be informed by different health ideologies, the development needs of the organisation, a wider social vision, or the political priorities and agenda of the day. These are not necessarily shared or coherent. Ensuring that your view of the purpose of your activity can be reconciled with organisational goals requires engagement with all those to whom you may be accountable: fellow professionals, managers, policy actors, the public and individual patients.

(3) **Strategy**

A strategy reflects the capacity and process for realising objectives. It is defined with reference to the fundamental goals or purposes of an organisation and the changes (or anticipated changes) in the environment which may affect its ability to achieve those goals (Waterman et al., 1980). Mintzberg argued for the separation of planning and strategy on the grounds that planning alone cannot deal adequately with uncertainty and discontinuity[3]. Strategy should be flexible, responsive and emergent. Assessing strategic performance is therefore as much about assessing the development and maintenance of the relationships that allow strategy to be effectively formed and implemented, as about meeting planning targets. For the stakeholder organisation, the characteristics of which NHS organisations are increasingly

---

[2] This approach to strategic management was developed in the early 1990s by Kaplan and Norton (1996).

[3] Mintzberg (1988). See also Morton (1998) p. 187 for processual perspectives on this subject.

expected to display through their openness and inclusiveness, a responsive strategy means more than simply looking at the external environment (by using PEST[4] analyses or other tools) but 'engaging in systematic dialogue with the networks of stakeholder relationships' (Wheeler & Sillanpää, 1997, p. 132). Collaborative relationships are thus an important aspect of organisational capacity and hence subject to performance assessment. For health professions this is a radical change.

(4) **Planning is the operationalising of strategy**

Detailed plans give rise to targets, indicators and a timeline to monitor progress. Performance is about meeting these targets which, at least in the UK, have tended to proliferate in number. Indicators are meant to be attributable (i.e. not merely reflect exposure to a co-variable), important, avoid perverse incentives, robust, responsive to change, measurable and readily available[5]. This is not always the case. Leadership, strong collaborative relations with partners, and collaboration with policy actors (and between policy actors) are needed to ensure that indicators are a positive developmental tool.

(5) **The definition of value will also shape our account of performance**

Is something worth doing? Does it enhance performance or is it wasteful? Concerns about performance are greatest when what is seen as being of long-term importance, of value to patients, or clinically desirable is not seen as contributing to performance, and may even be seen as detrimental to performance. Money is a reductionist measure of value when used in isolation. The move to 'best value contracting' in public services from more narrowly financially oriented compulsory competitive tendering illustrates that there is more to value than price. Layard, drawing on recent work on the economics of happiness, has pointed out that happiness has not increased in the UK over the last 50 years despite a significant rise in Gross Domestic Product. A strict utilitarian approach to health policy, informed by a good understanding of what actually enhances happiness, might, he argues, set some very different priorities[6]. The desire for a wider definition of value is also seen in approaches to valuing companies. Measures of intellectual, emotional, relational and human capital are now proposed to complement financial indicators (Roos & Jacobsen, 1999). Practical implications of this for health professions might include the extent to which time spent on research, interprofessional education, or building partnerships is adequately factored in performance assessment. They are valuable and strengthen an organisation, but the financial dividends are not necessarily realised in the short term.

---

[4] The acronym PEST is used to describe salient features of the external environment. It stands for Political, Economic, Social and Technological factors.
[5] From a consultation document on high level performance indicators (NHS Executive, 1998) quoted in Greenhalgh and Eversley (1999) p. 16.
[6] Layard (2003). A greater investment in mental health is one consequence that he suggests.

The account of performance implicit in the national planning and priorities guidance goes some way to addressing these issues. The basic framework can be traced back to the White Paper: *A First Class Service: Quality in the New NHS*, which sets out six areas of performance: health improvement (reducing inequality), fair access, effective delivery, efficiency, patient experience and health outcomes (Secretary of State for Health, 1998). A similar model applies for social services departments, which establishes five domains of performance: national priorities and strategic objectives; cost and efficiency; effectiveness of service delivery and outcomes; quality of services for users and cares; and fair access (Social Services Performance Assessment Framework Indicators 2002–2003, p. 21). The influence of a number of theoretical models of quality can be seen in these policies including, for example, the Donabedian distinction between structure, process and outcome[7], or Argyris and Schon's distinction between 'doing things right' (effectiveness, efficiency, respect, safety and timeliness) and 'doing the right thing' (appropriateness, availability and efficacy)[8].

Another model is the three 'E's of efficiency, economy and effectiveness. Here performance is principally understood in terms of:

- Volume of output (assessed by reference to targets)
- Finance (monitoring and controlling expenditure through audit, purchasing and managerial approaches to efficiency)
- Quality of output (assessed though clinical audit and governance with reference to service frameworks and regulatory requirements)

These may exist in some tension for professionals: if finance, for example, is a constant factor there may be some trade-offs between increasing the quality of care provided and increasing the number of patients treated. Both can be achieved, but not always. The power to determine what counts as performance, and what should be seen as acceptable levels of performance within this definition, conveys significant influence within a health service. This is one of the reasons why such concepts as quality can come to be treated with suspicion as an instrument of control rather than as a positive value.

What influences performance?

The case for collaboration rests on the link between relationships and performance. This link does not depend on any one particular account of performance. In this section we offer a summary of three ways in which collaboration and performance are linked, before considering a number of specific relational factors that influence performance.

---

[7] Donabedian (1980), generally regarded as the godfather of this subject area.
[8] Argyris and Schon (1978). See also the discussion of this in Greenhalgh and Eversley (1999) p. 10.

First, collaboration can improve performance. As any professional involved in admission or discharge arrangements is all too well aware, performance is affected by what other people and organisations do. This applies not just to the performance of a whole system, but also to individuals. We do not work in isolation. Collaboration is needed to ensure that interaction with, and dependency on, other people and agencies, enhances performance. A hospital's ability to meet waiting list targets, for example, may be influenced by the ability of local social services to provide residential or nursing care for elderly people. The orthopaedic surgeon's ability to treat an elderly person may depend, in part, on the ability of others to manage circulatory and respiratory problems. Health agencies may be held accountable (with others) for public health goals over which they have little or no direct influence. It is therefore important that one is clear about which relationships will impact on areas of performance for which one is held accountable, as well as recognising whose performance may be critically affected by one's own actions.

Second, managing performance should be a collaborative endeavour within the context of a shared commitment to improvement. The experience is sometimes rather different: of a distant relationship where collecting performance data diverts resources from other activities and is not a useful tool for personal or local service development. Seeking a more collaborative approach has implications for a wide range of internal relationships – such as those within executive boards, within and between professions, and between clinicians and managers – as well as the external relationships of scrutiny and inspection. Good governance enables early identification of problems so that remedial action can be taken[9]. The drive for quality improvement in business has focused heavily on the contribution of workplace relationships to create the feedback mechanisms which quickly identify problems and propose (and implement) solutions[10]. The Higgs report into the effectiveness of non-executive directors in the NHS emphasised that 'this lies as much in behaviours and relationships as in structures and processes' and that 'these relationships should be characterised by a spirit of partnership and mutual respect' (Higgs, 2003, para. 63).

Independent assessment is needed as well, but this should, as the following chapter demonstrates, still be linked to a concern for development. Thus, in a recent review of the inspection function in the UK, it was concluded that 'checking compliance with rules and regulations has long been superseded by today's needs for inspection to be a catalyst for better local leadership, confidence, creativity and innovation'[11]. Forms of inspection where targets are owned and

---

[9] In the UK the Audit Commission has recently looked at the contribution of corporate governance to improvement and trust in public services (Audit Commission, 2003).
[10] Dr W. Edwards Deming is widely regarded as one of the early leading proponents of this approach. Deming (2000) explores the implications for management.
[11] Office for Public Service Reform (2003) page 2. This built on the work of an earlier report by the Public Services Productivity Panel (Byatt & Lyons, 2001).

plans agreed with inspectors were seen as an important part of achieving this. As Chapter four has shown, the nature and quality of relationships is an important factor in identifying potential breakdowns and resolving poor performance. Openness about weakness in performance needs supportive relationships of mutual trust. Critical independence is also needed, and the challenge is to develop forms of collaborative relationship which neither lapse into collusive complacency, nor introduce such a degree of distance that concerns are not raised, or cannot be discussed effectively. In answering the question: 'How do executive and non-executive personnel ensure that they establish a professional and productive relationship that enables them to work together in partnership, but also allows them to hold, or to be held, to account?' the Audit Commission concluded that 'the key is that intangible asset: trust' (Audit Commission, 2003, para. 133).

Third, the process of monitoring performance is always likely to distort activity and can create incentives that undermine collaborative relationships as well as promoting them. Targets are indicators, not detailed accounts of all that is important. Data can be massaged and manipulated to create a misleading impression. Resources can be diverted from local and clinical priorities to meet the targets of those whose accountability carries more punch. Individual success can be pursued to the detriment of the wider and greater good of the service. Some responses to waiting time targets in the UK have been a particular cause of professional concern, including, for example, the fear that decisions on treatment might not always be based on clinical need – particularly if prioritising some routine cases can lead to a more rapid reduction in waiting times. The pressures are real: sustaining collaboration in such a context is not always easy, but may in fact be the route towards a better approach. Making a service, or system, the focus of performance management is intended to reduce the dangers, but divergent individual accountabilities can still easily come to the fore. Where there are significant rewards or penalties at stake the dangers of distortion are greater.

There are, of course, many factors which influence performance. The evidence base in some areas is, however, limited (Pearson, 2003). Factors such as market forces, performance related pay, investment, regulation and restructuring might be the focus. Whilst recognising that many variables are involved we will concentrate here on some of the key relationship factors which make the case for collaboration. The following is an illustrative rather than exhaustive analysis.

(1) **Organisational culture**
    The overall importance of relational factors is highlighted in a study of 850 high-performing organisations by the Talent Foundation (2001). This considered seven factors which distinguished award-winning companies which continued to perform highly, from those where performance had deteriorated. These were balancing today and tomorrow, innovating flexibly, sharing knowledge via relationships, seeing potential in staff, motivating

through valuing, building skills through informal learning and leading by cultivating. Each of these has implications for relationships within the organisation. Perhaps of particular note is the importance of learning and leadership style. Chapter four has illustrated the price of failing to learn and empower staff. The positive dividends can be equally significant. Top performers were found to be twice as likely to have strong relationships in place at all levels of the organisation (Talent Foundation, 2001, p. 14).

(2) **Governance and leadership**
The importance of this is emphasised by the Audit Commission in their view of the importance of achieving balance between a number of factors which are summarised in Table 5.2.

> 'Even organisations with good leaders, robust systems and processes, and those that are aware of the public's need, can still take wrong decisions, or be knocked off kilter by external forces. But with the right balance, they are both less likely to do so and to be able to recover more quickly if they do' (Audit Commission, 2003, para. 115). This is seen as part of the process of 'enabling discussions about governance to move on from a focus on compliance and preventing failure towards improvement'. Health and social care professions will need to find ways of striking the right balance in all their accountability relationships if they are to enhance performance.

(3) **Partnering**
The commissioning or purchasing relationship can be viewed in partnership terms. This is a richer relationship than competitive contracting based on price alone, and can facilitate improvements in cost, efficiency and quality. Xerox, for example, estimated that the lack of trust in their buyer/supplier

Table 5.2 Achieving balance in governance.

Requirement to balance	Possible response
Direction and negotiation	Upholding non-negotiable objectives and winning support for strategies
Rigidity and flexibility	High performers may focus more flexibly on outcomes: new organisations and poor performers may be required to pay more attention to basic systems and processes
Central direction and local autonomy	Balanced through setting timescales if not priorities
Key priorities and diverse responsibilities	Immediate demands must be balanced with continuing responsibilities
Compliance and creativity	Balancing improvement and assurance
Caution and ambition	Seeking realistic ambition, linked to capacity
Support and sanctions	Learning, in the context of both good and poor performance, requires a balance of both
Short and longer-term actions	Some timeframes are imposed, others adopted: clarity is needed about both pace and objectives

Audit Commission (2003) para. 115.

relationships cost them seven cents in the dollar[12]. Partnering has been promoted in the construction industry to save both construction costs and time (Egan, 1998). Preferred suppliers can develop a better understanding of their customers' needs and proactively identify ways in which processes can be improved and costs saved to mutual advantage. In this context, assessing performance is more than contractual enforcement (although that bottom line remains). It is about recognising that both parties benefit from improved performance and can help each other in that process. This is of particular relevance in commissioning health care, where there is little choice of provider, and therefore few options in terms of developing alternative collaborative relationships. At the heart of this relationship is a recognition that both purchaser/commissioner and provider of a service are seeking to serve patients. This can be lost sight of in the midst of the demands of a contracting process or the pressures of organisational survival. In reviewing one such relationship we found that too little time was taken to develop a shared strategic framework, and to understand each other's needs and priorities in the light of this. Identifying the times of the year when such an investment of time could be made, and would be most useful, was a simple but important step forward.

(4) **Expectations**
Performance responds to the expectations expressed in each of the six key relationships. Where too little is expected poor performance may not be challenged. Where expectations are unrealistic dissatisfaction may set in. Effective performance management is aided by appropriate expectations which do not neglect an account of the responsibilities that may accompany them. Setting expectations is an educative, and thus relational process and should not be a purely political and media driven process. It is a relationship in which health and social care professions should be active participants.

(5) **Civil society**
A final area for consideration is the impact of civil society on performance, both through the nature of demands that arise as well as through the potential of civil society to be an effective resource enhancing partner in provision[13]. Public health, relationally defined, will impact on performance. This may, for example, be a result of lower levels of social support or the consequence of different lifestyles. The quality of care for many vulnerable people depends on the contribution of family and informal carers. Without their practical contribution, as well as their advocacy role, the demands on health and social care providers would be much greater. The concern for long-term sustainable performance, accordingly, points towards health agencies seeing themselves as collaborative partners in civic renewal.

---

[12] Carlisle (1999) illustrates the financial benefits from a number of industries.
[13] Campbell and Wood (1999) in a report for the UK Health Development Agency look at the links between social capital and health.

Lessons for key relationships

What, then, are the implications for the key professional relationships of a broad and inclusive account of performance which gives due recognition to the range of relationships which influence its practice? Performance is, most importantly, a product of personal motivation – the desire to do a good job and to address health needs. What motivates may vary between individuals: for some people it will primarily be internally (and ethically) directed whilst for others it will be more shaped by external factors. An organisational culture where individuals take the initiative to identify improvements and seek high standards is very different from one where minimal compliance with externally imposed standards is the norm.

Performance is not, however, purely a personal concern. Each individual's performance, and the performance of the teams and organisations of which they are part, is of concern to others. The differing nature and extent of these concerns is partially a reflection of different patterns of health and social care relationships, but also shapes these patterns. The experience of performance management in the UK, which remains significantly influenced by centrally directed polices and plans, is very different to that in, for example, Peru where, as described in Chapter three, local communities have much greater influence over health and social care provision. The case for collaboration in these relationships is twofold: to create the kind of relationships within which the definition of performance includes the interests and concerns of both parties, and to create the kinds of relationships that enhance performance.

Own profession

Self-regulation has long been seen as a defining feature of what it means to be a profession and, until comparatively recently, has been the principal, even sufficient, assurance of quality[14]. The relationship with fellow professionals is still of great importance. They have a responsibility to ensure that individual performance meets certain standards. This may be at the time of seeking to become a member of the profession; continuing membership of the profession through appraisal, or in response to complaints about negligent or unethical performance. Research is peer-reviewed, recognising that those working in the same or related fields are best qualified to assess the quality of research and writing.

Clinical audit and governance create mechanisms by means of which members of the same profession can monitor each other's professional practice. This changes the dynamic of the relationship. No longer are professionals solely responsible for their own performance, vouchsafed by others at key moments. The relationship with fellow professionals is now increasingly set in an organisational context with professionals accountable for the performance of a service, not just their own personal role. The relationship, and the concern for performance,

---

[14] For historical accounts of the place of professions in society see, for example, O'Day (2000) and Perkins (2002).

thus takes on added significance. They may be judged by the performance of colleagues. Weaknesses in their performance (for example with respect to prescribing) may impact on the ability to develop new services for their patients. As Chapter six will explore, this can, and should, be viewed positively as an opportunity for professional development and improving service quality if this relationship is seen as a learning environment.

The link between learning, collaboration and performance is captured in the role of GPs with a special interest (GPWSI) promoted in NHS plan (DoH, 2000). The sharing of learning within (and now increasingly between) professions has long been seen as central to the advancement of health care. The GPWSI role is seen as one mechanism for enabling specialist experience to be accessible to a wider range of practitioners in such areas as mental health and drugs treatment. The Royal College of General Practitioners recommended that evidence of collaborative practice should be required in accrediting practices, practitioners and services for the GPWSI role (RCGP, undated).

Other professions

The collaborative responsibility for service provision brings other professions into the equation. Increasing specialisation has been pursued as one approach to improving performance, but this now needs to be coupled with greater integration of services. The role of other professions in maintaining and improving performance may be based on the collaborative relationships that arise from working with them to provide health care. As Chapter four has discussed, the intra-professional relationship of anaesthetist and surgeon should have allowed low survival rates in paediatric cardiac surgery to be properly investigated in Bristol.

If clinical governance has been the process for engaging people of the same profession in monitoring performance, clinical and public health networks have been important mechanisms for engaging other professions. The concern for performance can easily focus on the vertical relationships of service 'silos'; networks allow the horizontal relationship to be considered. This can take many forms including, for example, that between general practitioner and specialist around treatment and diagnosis. Specialists are in a good position to monitor how effectively diseases such as cancer are being diagnosed, and to support improvement by feedback or use of telemedicine. Generalists, acting as patients' advocates, can monitor whether specialist treatment is meeting their patients' needs. Working with other professions around patient pathways can identify opportunities for improvement. The benefits, for example, in terms of access to care, can be significant.

As health care management has developed as a profession, this has become one of the key interprofessional relationships concerned with performance. This relationship has not always been rooted in a strong sense of common purpose, with different accountabilities creating tension. These differences are summarised in a recent article:

'The clinician's traditional values are professional autonomy, the focus on individual patients, the desire for self-regulation and the role of evidence-based practice. In contrast, managers' values are the emphasis on populations, the need for public accountability, the preoccupation with systems and the allocation of resources'.

(BMJ (2003) p. 609 quoted in Audit Commission (2003) p. 12.)

Collaboration requires both professional groups to accept both sets of accountability, even if their work is oriented to one more than the other.

The role of other professions can be more distant than working together, albeit still within the context of shared organisational accountability. So, for example, in a university context staff from other departments provide a more independent view in research assessment exercises and can also improve performance by sharing learning and experience. The informed and supportive 'outsider' can sometimes ask the necessary tough and searching questions which challenge assumptions. The recent accounting scandals in the business sector (Enron and Worldcom being two of the most widely publicised examples) raised concerns that accountancy as a profession had lost the proper balance between a supportive role with the client (often linked to lucrative consulting work), and their relationship with shareholders, regulators and the wider public. Too close a collaboration in business improvement through consulting was perceived to limit the degree of independence that auditing requires. Too little involvement with the business, however, may limit the ability to advise on putting proper controls in place and to understand the full complexity of an individual business' workings. This suggests that a strong professional culture, particularly with regard to its ethics, is an important factor in getting these relationships right.

Partners

Three aspects of the relationship with partners are relevant to performance. Performance may be assessed by partners, particularly where a contractual commitment is monitored. An example is given in Table 5.1 which includes the commitment of a commissioning organisation 'to satisfy ourselves that key providers are demonstrating quality improvements in their services' (Cambridge PCT, 2003, p. 26). Performance may be affected by the quality of partner organisations' work and their capacity. Or there may be a collective responsibility for performance within a formal partnership structure.

Commissioning organisations may be held accountable for the quality of health care provision and so assessed by the performance of providers over whom they have limited influence or control. Health care organisations may also depend upon the work of other agencies, and their performance may be adversely affected by the knock-on consequences of a partner organisation's financial difficulties or weaknesses in performance. One example in the UK was a dispute between an ambulance trust and a hospital accident and emergency department. The latter was struggling to meet its targets on trolley waits and so was delaying formally admitting patients. This delayed the paramedics' turnaround time and so put pressure on their ability to meet response time targets. A more widespread example is the impact on hospitals of difficulties in funding and providing residential and nursing care for elderly people. The resulting 'bed-blocking' reduces the available capacity to meet other targets. It may prove worthwhile investing in partner organisations' capacity where this will improve one's own performance. This may be aided by strategic investment from policy actors who may be better placed to invest for the benefit of the system.

The problems of managing the interaction of performance have encouraged the promotion of a stronger sense of collective responsibility between partners. A few years ago we reviewed the relationship between managers of hostels for homeless people and local authority departments. In one case local authority housing and social service directors talked proudly of their collaborative relationship. Life on the ground was rather different. The housing department had no responsibility to fund accommodation for someone who was declared 'intentionally homeless'. The hostel manager (in a local authority run hostel) was required to evict them even if she knew the social services department had no effective provision in place for the children affected. Vulnerable people could easily fall through the cracks in the system. The tired response of the manager was: 'I don't have the capacity to manage other people's failures'. Coping – emotionally, physically and financially – required distancing from outcomes. When resources are scarce there is the danger that partners can compete either to avoid responsibility for provision, or in dividing up the available funding. With no strong shared accountability for outcomes, and strict assessment of their own narrowly defined performance, people suffer. This is the environment that breeds the service failures described in Chapter four.

Policy actors

Policy actors can influence collaboration by ensuring that their performance assessment role fosters rather than undermines collective accountability. In the UK this was signalled by the introduction of the phrase 'a duty of partnership' in early modernising policies (Secretary of State for Health, 1997). It can be promoted by national service frameworks, with a 'tsar' appointed to provide unifying leadership and progress on implementation subject to review[15]. Creating new structures and strategic processes have also been important reforming tools for health policy actors. The nature of politics does not, however, sit easily with responsibility for complex adaptive systems, where the link between intervention and outcome is uncertain and hard to predict. Where the levers of power are limited, influencing the system too often appears prescriptive and coercive.

The relationship between health professions and policy actors is not always seen and experienced in terms of collaboration, or sometimes only in the negative sense of traitorous cooperation with an occupying power. There is, of course, a recognition of the need for collaboration in the sense that political promises of delivery can only be honoured through the work of health professions. Where, however, reform is seen as the key to improved delivery, this sense of collabor-

---

[15] See, for example, the Commission for Heath Improvement review of the Cancer National Service Framework (CHI, 2001).

ation can be obscured by competing claims to be advocates of the public interest. Health professions claim to defend the public against the ravaging impact of misguided policies, while policy actors claim to work for the public interest against the vested interests of 'dinosaur' professions.

The dynamics of the performance relationship between professions and policy actors has implications for the relationship between professions and the public. The challenge is to construct some sense of collaborative shared accountability to the public between professions and policy actors, a sense of both working for the common good. Until reform is truly seen as a collaborative endeavour between government and services, with both trusting each other's motives, commitment and objectives, then ensuring and driving performance risks being coercive. For professions this means accepting responsibility and being trusted by both public and policy actors as effective guardians of quality. In a workshop exploring public health relationships one health authority chief executive saw this as part of her leadership responsibility. She described this in terms of providing 'air cover': shielding those below from overly intrusive performance management by accepting responsibility for the delivery of outcomes, and putting her head over the parapet to relieve the need for those above to be too closely involved. Without trust, justified by the experience of effective performance, such relationships are hard to sustain.

Public

The policy theme of local resource management creates an opportunity for greater public involvement in the scrutiny of services. As is the case with scrutiny by policy actors, performance is most likely to be improved where there is a collaborative aspect to this relationship. Local government scrutiny remains underdeveloped in the UK, though the opportunities represented by local government oversight committees should strengthen this role (Centre for Public Scrutiny, 2002). Internationally, higher levels of local authorities' co-payments give them a greater stake in performance[16]. Health agencies also need to develop collaborative relationships with the public and community groups in order to meet public health goals. This collaborative relationship can also have development benefits, where engaging communities in evaluation increases and empowers their ownership of services. The link between public involvement and community development is more evident in such countries as Chile and Peru[17] than in the UK.

Patients

Patients have a strong and legitimate interest in performance: it is their well-being that is at stake. The patient as consumer influences performance through the exercise of choice, with the financial consequences of these choices creating performance incentives (although poor performers can be put under greater pressure through loss of income). Where the patient is an empowered partner in health care, this collaborative relationship can enhance performance through taking greater

---

[16] The implications of this for local health care relations in the Philippines are discussed on pages 49–50.
[17] See the discussion in Chapter six, as well as previous discussion in Chapters one and three.

responsibility for their own health, aiding diagnosis, better compliance with treatment and helping to ensure that real needs are met[18]. Carers and advocates are also important partners and it is worth investing in their care skills. As well as the direct provision of care they can provide quick feedback on poor care, enabling remedial action, and can serve as a focus of integration in a fragmented system. Policy is driving the organisational relationships which can support improved delivery of health outcomes. This needs to be seen by health and social care professionals as a better context for the relationship with the patient, not a substitute for it. Patients use and rely on services, but at their most vulnerable they need the care of the individual professionals who comprise that service.

Lessons

Performance satisfies the demands of relationships and is achieved through relationships. It must be rooted in a clear sense of purpose, what is truly valuable, and develop relationships that build strategic capacity. Organisations and services are, increasingly, the main focus of performance assessment. What needs to be done cannot be done alone. Modernising policies shift the location and structures of accountability, which have greater complexity in the context of integrated cross boundary partnerships. In this context professions must consider how each of the six key relationships can enhance their own performance and that of others, and seek to develop a performance assessment process that is collaborative and developmental. This concern for development is the focus of the next chapter.

Bibliography

Argyris, C. & Schön, D. (1978) *Organisational Learning: a Theory of Action Perspective.* Addison Wesley, London.

Audit Commission (2003) *Corporate Governance: Improvement and Trust in Public Services.* Audit Commission, London.

Byatt, I. & Lyons, M. (2001) *Public Services Productivity Panel Report: Role of External Review in Improving Performance.* HM Treasury, London.

Cambridge City Primary Care Trust (2003) *Local Delivery Plan 2003–2006.* Cambridge City Primary Care Trust, Cambridge.

Campbell, C. & Wood, R. (1999) *Social Capital and Health.* Health Education Authority, London.

Carlisle, J. (1999) *Cooperation Works But it's Hard Work.* John Carlisle Partnerships, Sheffield.

Centre for Public Scrutiny (2002) *The Scrutiny Map.* IDEA Publications, London.

Commission for Heath Improvement (2001) *NHS Cancer Care in England and Wales: National Service Framework Assessments No. 1.* Commission for Health Improvement, London.

Commission for Health Improvement (2002) *Final Performance Indicators for Primary Care Trusts.* Commission for Health Improvement, London.

---

[18] A renewed interest in the therapeutic relationship is seen, for example, in Dixon and Sweeney (2000).

Deming, W. (2000) *Out of the Crisis*. MIT Press, Massachusetts.

Department of Health (2000) *The NHS Plan: a Plan for Investment, a Plan for Reform*. Department of Health, London.

Department of Health (2002) *Improvement, Expansion and Reform: the Next Three Years. Priorities and Planning Framework 2003–2006*. Department of Health, London.

Dixon, M. & Sweeney, K. (2000) *The Human Effect in Medicine: Theory, Research and Practice*. Radcliffe Medical Press, Abingdon.

Donabedian, A. (1980) *Explorations in Quality Assessment and Monitoring Vol. 1: Definition of Quality and Approaches to Assessment*. Health Administration Press, Ann Arbor Michigan.

Egan, J. (1998) *Rethinking Construction*. Department of Trade and Industry, London.

Greenhalgh, T. & Eversley, J. (1999) *Quality in General Practice*. King's Fund, London.

Higgs, D. (2003) *Review of the Role and Effectiveness of Non-executive Directors*. Department of Trade and Industry, London.

Kaplan, R. & Norton, D. (1996) *Balanced Scorecard: Translating Strategy into Action*. Harvard Business School Press, Boston.

Layard, R. (2003) *Happiness: Has Social Science a Clue?* Lionel Robbins Memorial Lectures.

Mintzberg, H. (1988) *The Rise and Fall of Strategic Planning*. Prentice Hall, Hemel Hempstead.

Morton, C. (1998) *Beyond World Class*. Macmillan Business, Basingstoke.

O'Day, R. (2000) *Professions in Early Modern England*. Pearson Education, Harlow.

Pearson, R. (2003) *Recruiting and Developing an Effective Workforce in the NHS*. Institute for Employment Studies, Sussex.

Perkins, H. (2002). *The Rise of Professional Society*. Routledge, London.

Royal College of General Practitioners (undated) *Accreditation, Appraisal and Revalidation*. Advisory group on drug misuse, London.

Roos, G. & Jacobsen, K. (1999) Management in a complex stakeholder organisation: a case study. *Monash Mt Eliza Business Review*, **2**, (1) pp. 83–93.

Secretary of State for Health (1997) *The New NHS: Modern, Dependable*. HMSO, London.

Secretary of State for Health (1998). *A First Class Service: Quality in the New NHS*. HMSO, London.

Social Services Inspectorate (2002) *Social Services Performance Assessment Framework Indicators 2002–2003* p. 21. Department of Health, London.

Talent Foundation (2001) *Seven Factors for Business Success*. Talent Foundation, London.

Waterman, R., Peters, T. & Philips, J. (1980) The Seven S Framework. In: *The Strategy Process* (ed. Quinn, J. & Mintzberg, H.) pp. 309–14 Prentice Hall, Englewood Cliff New Jersey.

Wheeler, D. & Sillanpää, M. (1997) *The Stakeholder Corporation*. Pitman Publishing, London.

Further Reading

Edwards, N., Marshall, M., McLellan, A. & Abassi, K. (2003) Doctors and managers: a problem without a solution? No, a constructive dialogue is emerging. *British Medical Journal*, **326**, 609–10.

NHS Executive (1998) *The New NHS – Modern, Dependable: a National Framework for Assessing Performance. Attachment C (EL(98)4)*. NHS Executive, Leeds.

Office for Public Service Reform (2003) *Inspecting for Improvement: Developing a Customer Focused Approach*. Office for Public Service Reform, London.

6 Development

Context

In this chapter we examine the development agenda around collaboration. Our justification for doing so is straightforward. Development is considered to be of importance since, as we shall see, it is often health and social care professionals who are charged with the responsibility for ensuring that collaborative policies and directives are put into place. Alongside regulation and performance management, development is one of the three practical imperatives for collaboration.

Globally, as Chapter three illustrated, numerous examples of good practice in interprofessional and inter-agency collaboration exist. Moreover, as described in Chapter one, collaboration is a key element of modern health and social care organisations and professions. Internationally, collaboration has become more important than ever, with the shift that has taken place during the last 20 years towards providing health and social care within the community wherever possible, rather than within institutions. Whilst globally the approaches adopted to facilitate greater collaboration vary, the drivers behind the push towards collaboration and the integration of services are similar. There is international recognition that the integration of services and collaboration of organisations and professionals within them leads to more effective and efficient services for the client (WHO, 2000; Mur & van Raak, 2003). Furthermore, collaboration is deemed a necessary response to the world's ageing population. The conviction – based on much belief and some evidence – is that collaboration helps each individual profession to deliver a more appropriate and valuable service. The aim of providing a seamless service to users relies heavily on the collaboration of individuals and agencies in order for it to be realised. The development of interprofessional education itself is a major response to these collaborative and partnership arrangements now favoured throughout much of the world.

Purpose

This chapter will identify developments within interprofessional learning that aim to facilitate increased collaboration. The chapter will also describe some of the examples of good practice in collaboration in service developments and delivery arrangements. In addition, the development agendas driving collaboration through innovative curriculum design and service developments internationally arising from modernisation policies, and how these change the nature of 'development' will be explored. This chapter draws on international literature detailing developments in interprofessional education (IPE) as well as the development of integrated services, on relevant conference material, data collected during fieldwork as part of the 12 country case study outlined in Chapter one (p. 5), and current UK and international policy documents including relevant WHO declarations and guidelines.

The development agenda

Collaboration is a relatively recent strategy to feature prominently in health policy across the globe. It is fundamentally connected to the modernisation of health and social care systems that has taken place predominantly over the last ten years. Almost everywhere is starting from the basis of different organisational cultures, education and training, professional cultures and priorities, all of which need to be developed in order to facilitate collaboration. However, developing collaboration (and its preconditions) is widely recognised to be difficult. Yet an examination of the number of policies and educational and service initiatives based upon a collaborative model, both in the UK and internationally, demonstrates a firm commitment to and belief in the efficacy of collaboration. The collaboration agenda, it seems, has been adopted wholesale by countries with modernising health systems. It is an act of faith.

   Given that the enhancement of patient care and the provision of a seamless service to users are fundamentally goals which all health and social care professionals would sign up to, and that professional and organisational collaboration is recognised as one of the key mechanisms by which this end can be achieved, it could be expected that the development agenda would go unchallenged. However, reliance on the public service ethos and claims to moral added-value are not enough to guarantee the successful adoption of collaborative practices. In particular, such an approach would show very little appreciation of the concerns professionals are themselves expressing about the future of individual professions. Nor does it recognise the confusion and uncertainty many feel about the long-term vision. Understandable as these concerns may be, an examination of the development of collaboration internationally, however, does not suggest the replacements of professionals with generic workers as is sometimes feared. Whilst new multi-skilled professional profiles which cross traditional professional boundaries are being created, for example Italy's Health and Social Care Workers (European Observatory on Health Care Systems, 2001) these new occupational roles are supplementing the traditional professions and usually acting as first point of contact workers (for example the development of Mental Health 'Gateway' workers to work in primary health care in England, as cited in Chapter three).

Whilst in practice informal collaboration between frontline workers has always existed, its formalisation and inclusion as a key strategy, to be adopted by the health and social care sectors per se and featuring extensively in policy, is a relatively recent phenomenon. Furthermore, professional bodies, such as the Royal College of General Practitioners (RCGP) in the UK and the US American Academy of Nurse Practitioners (AANP), have produced their own sets of standards relating to collaborative practice.

Levels of development

Collaboration requires development at three separate, yet interrelated levels:

(1) Personal development
(2) Organisational development
(3) Service development

An integrated service cannot be achieved unless organisations recognise the importance of working together and facilitate that collaboration through an organisational culture which promotes cooperation and flexibility in the development of new joint positions, shared systems across organisations, collective ownership and new collaborative management arrangements with joint accountability. However, organisational collaboration in health and social care is ultimately reliant upon the acceptance and ability of individual professionals within the organisation to work across traditional boundaries; hence the need to develop the skills and capacity of individuals to collaborate.

Responsibility for collaboration development

Development of collaborative practice is very often the responsibility of frontline services. Local agencies frequently recognise the need for collaboration and integration and respond accordingly, usually appointing a 'lead' organisation. This form of horizontal development relating to collaboration is a feature of modernising countries, which now rely less upon vertical top-down or bottom-up initiatives to lead the development process.

Integrated service delivery and collaboration of individuals and organisations necessarily relies on the ability and willingness of professionals to work together. Moreover, it is the professional who is often expected to implement integration policies and upon whose energies implementation relies. Professionalism ensures high standards but, in the past, has often led to power hierarchies. Collaboration seeks to maintain the interest in high standards whilst overcoming the power hierarchies and silos to achieve equality between professions and integration of high quality services.

Collaborative practice as a 'modern imperative'

Interprofessional collaboration is at the heart of modernisation reforms in the UK and globally. This is our starting point. The five key elements of modernisation were set out in Chapter one:

(1) Local resource management (or decentralisation)
(2) Governance (with new forms of independent regulation)
(3) Integration (based on cross boundary partnerships)
(4) Stewardship for public health (and thence community development)
(5) Quality (linking evidence based health care to choice and consumerism)

These represent a holistic approach to the planning and delivery of health and social care and have necessitated the introduction of a number of key policies and developments requiring collaboration across traditional professional boundaries. Not all of these policies have been top-down. Some have been developed in response to pioneering local practice in service planning and delivery as well as developments in educational curricula and practice.

This holistic approach demands the development of robust partnerships between health and social care, in particular, but also with the voluntary and independent sectors. In the UK such collaborations have been underpinned by duties of partnership. For example, the *Health and Social Care Act* (2001) placed a duty of partnership on health and social care organisations, building on measures such as the integration of service provision, pooled budgets for health and social care services and lead commissioning arrangements introduced in the *Health Act* (1999) to facilitate integrated working. One of many manifestations of this can be seen in the formulation of interprofessional executive committees to manage English primary care trusts (PCTs), which include representation from community-based health professionals, local authority social services departments, a lay person and health service managers. In Portugal, where traditionally health has been viewed as a 'gift', partnerships have traditionally been dependent on the State. However, the development of cross-sectoral collaborations saw the development of public-private partnerships in the 1990s, such as the Hospital Amadera Sintrez in Lisbon and the multi-professional Institute for Quality in Health Care at Coimbra.

Whilst in the UK the Health and Social Care Act duty binds all health and social care organisations to work in partnership these new duties have been used more innovatively in organisations with increased flexibilities and a remit for developing integrated services which respond to local needs. The 1998–2002 Health Action Zones (HAZs) in England may be regarded as one such example of an initiative employing dedicated actions to improve collaboration amongst all professionals and agencies within a locality, including the voluntary and independent sectors and community organisations. In this case, the aim of collaboration was to provide more appropriate services for vulnerable groups and neighbourhoods experiencing high levels of socio-economic disadvantage. As initiatives which seek to influence mainstream organisational practice with the results of new service innovations and successful projects, HAZs avoided many of the criticisms of prior one-off partnership projects which disappear once their 'special funding' runs out. HAZs have been just one of a number of policies within the UK which seek to tackle social exclusion and health inequalities through joined-up working (Wild, 2002). The largest strategy, impacting upon all local authorities, is the National Strategy for Neighbourhood Renewal (Social Exclusion Unit, 2001), a wide-ranging regeneration and social inclusion programme that incorporates initiatives such as the New Deal for Communities.

This emphasis on partnership working, or what Clarence and Painter (1998) have called the 'collaborative discourse' is a feature of many of the UK's health and social policies post-1997 and the election of a New Labour Government. A far from exhaustive number of examples are given in Box 6.1 below as an indication of the breadth of policy areas now requiring joint working in the UK.

In many countries partnership working has now been extended to include central government with joined-up government at the centre of collaborative efforts. This is exemplified in the UK through the establishment of the central Office for Public Services Reform with a remit of coordinating activities across Government departments.

This emphasis on collaboration as a key feature of policies seeking to modernise and improve health and social care services can be seen across the world. In developing countries it is often non-governmental organisations (NGOs) which take the lead in driving forward programmes for collaboration. For example, in Uganda NGOs have utilised pooled sector funding arrangements following the 1996 establishment of their National Panel for collaboration with Government. One of the early products of this was the unified regulatory framework for nurses and midwives, dental practitioners and allied health professionals, regardless of their employment status.

Developments in interprofessional education and training

The direct collaboration of trainee doctors with other professionals such as nurses and midwives, often in conjunction with community health workers trained in health promotion is an approach found at the universities of Gezira and Alazhari in the Sudan, amongst other places. Initiatives such as COME (Community Oriented Medical Education) place medical students in poor rural areas as a means of both improving the health care of local residents and demonstrating

---

Box 6.1   Post-1997 UK Policies, 'The Collaborative Discourse'.

- Local Strategic Partnerships (LSPs) as set out in the *NHS Plan* (2000) are partnerships at the local authority level with a remit for encouraging core public services to work together in conjunction with the voluntary sector, private sector and communities to help shape the delivery of services in the future.
- The *National Strategy for Neighbourhood Renewal* launched in 2001 aims to harness the support of all sectors within deprived areas and get them to work in partnership with local residents and community groups and support them in turning their neighbourhoods around.
- The *Saving Lives: Our Healthier Nation* White Paper (1999) set out how coordinated action is being taken across Government to promote overall population health status and reduce specific morbidities.
- The Department of the Environment Transport and the Regions' (1998) *Modern Local Government: In Touch with the People* sets out the need for all parts of Government to work together better if services provided at the local level are to be improved.
- Local Compacts were introduced in July 2000 by the Department of the Environment, Transport and the Regions to improve relations between local statutory bodies and voluntary agencies. They provide guidelines on how to establish agreed ways of working across multiple agencies.
- Care Trusts, announced in the *NHS Plan* (2000) are vehicles for the integration of health and social services and allow the delivery of all health and social services by a single organisation, where locally this model is considered most appropriate.
- Health Action Zones were established after 1997 to bring together all agencies who can make a difference in terms of health, i.e. NHS bodies, police forces, educational bodies, local authorities, private businesses, voluntary organisations, community organisations etc, in order to highlight the interdependence of all of these different agencies and the importance of working together.
- Children's Trusts, beginning in 2004, are new structures that will enable organisations to join together in voluntary partnerships to plan, commission, finance and deliver children's services.

---

the importance of interprofessional collaboration amongst health workers. All trainee health professionals study case management skills, laboratory skills and health education and nutritional counselling skills, which they utilise in their joint placements. Students acquire skills in identifying health problems and community health needs, planning and implementing health interventions. It is argued that such an approach fosters social accountability amongst professionals and results in a more integrated service for users (The Network Conference, Kenya, 2002).

At Western Cape University in South Africa a 'Shared Community-Based Practice' approach is being piloted, which uses primary health care principles to target the poorest areas via interprofessional programmes. This module applies across the faculty and incorporates students of medicine, physiotherapy and public health. Operating in the fourth year of their training the students provide a service as part of their community attachment as well as undertaking local research and needs analyses. At Marilia Medical School in Brazil collaborative practice takes the form of groups of 12 students (eight doctors and four nurses) along with two health professionals (a doctor and a nurse) joining Family Health Units. Within the unit each takes co-responsibility for ten families in terms of identifying their health needs, setting up health problems and encouraging their participation in interventions. Whilst at Ghent University in Belgium trainee health professionals collaborate with social work students on a one-year Community Oriented Primary Care project[1]. Developments in multi-professional education are taking place across the world and are recognised as key to delivering the modernisation agenda.

Development of others, not just ourselves

As Chapter two noted, collaboration is not simply about many separate professions staying the same, but working together. Collaboration requires a re-evaluation of what it means to be a professional. Professions are now required to act as agents of development for others. The UK NHS Expert Patients Programme (Department of Health, 2001a), which helps people living with long-term conditions maintain their health and improve their quality of life through their participation in self management courses, is an example of how this works in practice. Moreover, collaboration does not just mean within the development of a service or across professions. The new mindsets and behavioural changes collaboration demands, as discussed in Chapter one, mean that the development of others is an essential element of development. In essence, collaboration must be viewed as a participative process.

Drivers for collaboration

Health systems across the world are recognising the value of providing a seamless service in terms of, for example, rationalising operations, standardising service provision and improving the quality of the service provided to users. In Finland, for example, municipalities have integrated their political, health care and social

---

[1] The source for this material was formal presentations and informal discussions with participants at The Network Conference in Newcastle, Australia, October 2003.

care boards into fewer, but larger boards in an attempt to overcome equity problems within the system. Another key driver for collaboration amongst professionals and organisations to improve the integration of services are the risks resulting from disjointed services and a lack of collaboration, as detailed in Chapter four. Indeed, poor performance within the health system as a whole is recognised by the WHO as a challenge throughout the world that could be improved through the enhanced integration of health and social services.

The UK Government argues that collaboration is essential because problems like high levels of crime, low levels of educational attainment and poor health are related, or need to be solved using 'joined-up' thinking. Consequently, the solutions to these problems also need to work across sectors and traditional boundaries.

Collaboration at the local level is often a response to national guidance (for example, the UK's National Service Frameworks) recommending closer working relationships amongst all agencies involved in the provision of care to particular groups. Indeed, the development of cross-sectoral public health targets, exemplified by National Service Frameworks (NSFs), requires joint strategies across agencies and sectors and may be regarded as a key driver for collaboration. The integration of care and provision of better coordinated services at the heart of NSFs requires multi-agency and multi-professional collaboration. For such developments to be successful professional collaboration is required at all levels, from coordination across Government departments, the integration of strategic management across welfare sectors and collaboration by frontline staff at the point of service delivery.

Personal and ethical principles can also act as drivers for collaborative development. This may be expressed in the form of a public service ethos amongst individuals, the desire to provide an efficient and integrated service to users, and personal appreciation of the benefits of teamworking and inter-agency collaboration. Collaboration is also driven forward by clinical and care demand management. For example, care management, shared protocols, individual needs assessments, managed care and care pathways are all new practice concepts that require different approaches to patient care which are essentially based upon interprofessional collaboration. Clinical governance programmes also require the collaboration of different professions in delivering evidence-based quality improvements and in the monitoring of standards. Furthermore, many professional career paths now reflect these interprofessional practices and are based upon relationships of collaboration. As noted in Chapter five, the performance of professionals in responding to these requirements for new models of delivering patient care impacts directly upon the ability of professionals to participate in collaborative relationships with others.

Expert/professional drivers for collaboration may also be found at the national and primary care levels through such organisations as the Royal College of General Practitioners in the UK and the Portuguese Association of GPs (APMCG) in Portugal and internationally through organisations like the World Bank and World Health Organization. Furthermore, as Chapter four describes, investigations into malpractice have also emphasised how better collaboration could have averted some of these tragedies. Consequently, a re-evaluation of the traditional methods of training professionals has recognised the need for integration of the professions during their period of training. This integration has been to various degrees and at different levels of training, undergraduate, postgraduate and continuing professional development. In the UK the pre-registration common learning project, described in Chapter one, includes a programme in which up to 13 professional groups come together for the whole first year of their training to undertake a common foundation year. In addition, the introduction of an NHS University (NHSU) over the 2002–2005 period will see the provision of a wide range of curricula designed for more generically skilled health and social care workers. The NHSU will work in partnership with social services, voluntary, private and user organisations to deliver learning to facilitate a patient-centred service with the emphasis on teamwork and collaboration.

Integration in educational programmes across health and social care sectors is relatively well advanced in Finland. A three and a half year integrated vocational study programme has been established to educate multi-professional practice nurses. This is designed to give them competence in basic medical work, home help and social care tasks. Training to become a Specialist in General Medicine takes six years post-qualification including four years based in a health centre with strong social services and education links (Niskamen, 2002).

At the University of Newcastle, Australia, the emphasis is on education and service partnerships with, for example, a Joint Skills Centre in which doctors and allied health professionals learn general techniques together (communications, airways management, wound dressing etc.). In Natal University, South Africa, there are also generic Clinical Skills Laboratories for all disciplines in years one and two of their training.

At Londrina, in Brazil, the Active Ageing educational programme promotes multidisciplinary approaches to working with people over 65 years of age. Dentistry and medical students with a specialist interest in cardiovascular disease, neuropsychiatric disorders and cavity health, amongst other conditions, learn and teach together in the community through joint lectures, surveys of older people's own perceptions of health and through the provision of domiciliary support (The Network Conference, Australia, 2003).

Across the globe action research (Lewin, 1946) and problem-based learning have been found to be some of the most effective ways for different professionals to learn together. Action research rejects the notion of objectivity and the non-reciprocal relationship between researcher and researched, preferring, instead, to adopt the principle of 'promoting change' through research. Within action research collaboration between the researcher and the researched is essential, with the researched taking an active role in the whole research process from the initial planning through to reflections on and use of the research findings. The problem or patient-based learning (PBL) approach is a core element of the Maastricht University medical education curriculum which emphasises the importance of medical students solving real patients' problems, under the supervision of a more experienced health professional. Responsibility for patients as part of a team involved in patient care forms an important part of the assessment process[2]. The Maastricht model has a worldwide influence on teaching and learning in health care.

Service development

These educational developments are mirrored by service developments. For example, inter-sectoral and interprofessional collaboration have increased considerably during the 1990s in Finland. Emphasis on collaboration in the health and social care sectors, in particular, has now extended to include collaboration in other sectors within Finland, such as education and employment. In 45% of Finnish municipalities the administration of health and social care is combined, and integration at the primary care service delivery level is encouraged. The focus is on providing a seamless service to the patient. Care is organised at the municipal level, rather than within separate sectors. These developments in interprofessional learning taking place across the globe are essential if the collaborative behavioural changes necessary to deliver the modernisation agenda are to be realised[3].

The WHO identifies the importance of collaboration amongst a wide range of health and social care agencies as well as with the community. In Mexico the community is defined as key partner in the development of materials used to promote health. The community is also heavily involved in the provision of services in rural and marginalised communities. As we have noted in Chapter three, community members are employed as Community Health Workers (CHWs) who are trained to provide medication, simple diagnosis and carry out health promotion activities. Community health workers receive a small financial contribution from health centres and mostly work in the public health system. The majority of communities with more than 100 people have a local committee, which includes three lay people from the area. Usually female, one of these local people takes on responsibility for checking that health services are being delivered properly and that people are using them; the second has the same role but related to education, and a third has responsibility for social development within the locality (income generation etc.)[4].

There is a need to recognise the demands the development agenda places on partners. For example, where collaborative relationships are developed between the statutory and voluntary sector it is essential to acknowledge the differences in capacity which may exist. Partners must invest time and resources in building the

---

[2] See for example Scherpbier (2001) *The New Maastricht Curriculum: Best Evidence-Based Medical Education.*

[3] Finland field trip by Meads and Wild, 2003.

[4] Mexico field trip by Meads and Wild, 2003.

capacity of partners who are less well resourced or less able to collaborate on an equal basis[5].

Key collaborative relationships

Let us now consider what we can learn about our six key professional relationships for today's health and social care professionals from these examples of good practice around interprofessional collaborative practice and educational developments. We will highlight a new 'modernised' approach to development under each.

With own profession

Own professional status and standards remain important. Collaboration is reliant upon each individual profession feeling confident enough in its own status not to feel threatened by the increased demand and need to collaborate with other professions. Initiatives seeking to strengthen collaboration may well begin by assessing care pathways and individual profession's workloads. Such 'workforce planning' can be extremely beneficial to professions in making a case for employing more staff and for delegating responsibility to other professions to ease the workload burden. Consequently professional autonomy may be strengthened.

Furthermore, as may be demonstrated by the inclusion of a number of health and social care professionals on the Professional Executive Committees of NHS primary care trusts in the UK, individual professions are also taking on increased responsibility for management decisions around health care planning and resource allocation.

With other professions

Health and social care professionals are increasingly experiencing a change in their relationship with other professions within an organisation, within a locality, as well as across geographical boundaries. The development of new mechanisms for delivering services (especially the shift towards teamworking), along with the co-location of services requires much more interprofessional collaboration. Curricula developments around interprofessional education (IPE) seek to produce professionals with enhanced understanding of the roles and remits of other professions; more appropriate referrals to other services; increased respect for the work of other professions, and ultimately, relationships based on equality or, at least, equivalence.

---

[5] For a more detailed discussion of these issues see Shaw and Ashcroft (2002).

CAIPE is the UK centre of expertise in developing and promoting interprofessional education and learning as a means of facilitating collaborative practice. It is increasingly informing developments in interprofessional learning globally and has a membership of individuals and organisations from across the health, social care and education sectors, which includes statutory and voluntary organisations as well as user groups. CAIPE tracks policy and service developments relevant to interprofessional learning and shares these with its members. It plays an important role in relation to innovation in methods of development (and evaluation)[6], for example the Interactive Learning and Training the Trainers approaches. Each of these adopts a sequential and standards based approach rooted in the need first to facilitate better mutual understanding through the sharing of agendas and overcoming of prejudices between professionals. An acceptance of equivalence amongst the latter is fundamental, with different and diverse contributions being harnessed in support of the single all consuming aim of meeting patient or client need[7].

With new partners

Collaboration is not only across traditional professional boundaries but also, as Chapter two has indicated, encompasses an increased role for citizens and voluntary sector organisations. The development agenda recognises the need to work with all involved in health and social care including individuals, families and carers as well as the benefit of working with private and voluntary sector partners. Consequently, new accountability and performance management arrangements are required which take into account the need for joint ownership and shared responsibility. New partners may also require a considerable investment of resources, including time, capacity-building, financial resources and so on. The Joint Reviews, originally initiated by the Audit Commission in 1997, are now a standard exercise of the post-2003 Social Care Commission and its NHS counterpart. In such collaborations, with new partners, as recent research has demonstrated[8], there is a pressing need for highly skilled facilitation, and sometimes mediation, with third parties often finding themselves filling the voids left by statutory agency professionals; and becoming, in effect, directly accountable for the delivery of central development priorities.

With policy actors

Collaboration and interprofessional education means new organisational frameworks and new policy documents and drivers. Internationally, agencies such as

---

[6] For example see Meads *et al.* (2003) paper on a CAIPE action research project which sought to develop and review new health and social care partnerships in London, UK.

[7] For further details of these and other CAIPE programmes see Appendix A or email: admin@caipe. org.uk

[8] See, for example, Meads *et al.* (2003) for a decidedly chequered picture of collaboration between partners in London.

the WHO's *The Network: Towards Unity for Health* (the Network) organisation play a leading role in the development of collaborative practice and the educational developments required to underpin collaboration. For example, their last three annual conferences, in Brazil, Kenya and Australia respectively, have all sought to promote interprofessional education and share information and educational expertise across members who represent many different countries and continents. The focus on community-oriented preventive and primary health care in the education of health professionals promoted by the Network, and the many practical examples of this which have been provided at Network conferences has influenced curriculum development in a number of medical schools and led many to rethink their own practice.

Within the UK, the NHS Alliance, which defines itself as a 'value-based organisation', may be regarded as a champion of collaboration within health care services. The NHS Alliance is the organisational representation of primary care in the UK. Its members represent primary care organisations as well as individual professions and major organisations such as the Royal College of Nursing. Established in 1998 the NHS Alliance grew out of the Locality Commissioning movement which sought to develop a culture of collective working within the NHS and a commitment to equity. Based on the principles of equity, inclusiveness, cooperation and democracy, the NHS Alliance advocates multi-professional working as well as equal relationships with all involved in health, including patients and the public[9].

With public

The public are now recognised as key partners in the process of health care planning. Public involvement is seen globally as an essential element of the process of modernisation of health care systems. Whilst Peru's CLAS system of local health committees discussed in Chapters one and three may be regarded as a leading international example, within the UK public involvement is now promoted through a number of national bodies as well as featuring heavily in many of the health and social care policies introduced since 1997. The organisation Voice was established to allow the public as citizens, rather than as patients, to comment on and influence the development of health services. Voice, as a group of specialist staff with public participation skills, works with communities to support and promote community involvement in local decision making. At the national level: the Commission for Patient and Public Involvement in Health was set up to monitor patient and public involvement across the health service. Within the *NHS Plan* (Secretary of State for Health, 2000) the UK Government also announced its intention to develop a Citizens Council to provide

---

[9] The NHS Alliance was formed in 1996–97 as a deliberate reaction against what was seen as the overweening, self-interested influence of the uni-disciplinary National Association of GP Fundholders, with the explicit aim of being interdisciplinary and, in particular, much more inclusive of local managers.

guidance to the National Institute for Clinical Excellence (NICE) in its decisions on treatments.

With patients

Patients are now recognised within health policy in modernising countries as legitimate partners in the process of health care decision making as well as in the management of their own care, as demonstrated by the introduction of initiatives such as the Expert Patients Programme. IPE and resulting service developments should result in enhanced relationships with patients and the ability to view needs holistically. Development of 'one-stop shops' for many health and social services reduces duplication and provides enhanced service to users. Development of shared patient records and other IT developments are a current priority in many modernising health systems[10]. The increased role of patients in their own care (and the public in the NHS and health more generally) can be seen within the UK in Government documents with titles such as *Patient and Public involvement in the new NHS* (Department of Health, 1999). It can also be seen in the establishment of a number of forums within which patient participation is expected to occur e.g. Patient Participation Groups within general practice, the requirement placed on PCTs to facilitate patient and public involvement, and in the fact that each primary care trust and NHS trust had to establish its own Patients' Forum as the arena within which local patients could participate. Patients' Forums were established to monitor the standards of care received and have powers to inspect all aspects of the work of NHS trusts (Department of Health, 2001b). Furthermore the Government established Patient Advocacy and Liaison Services (PALS) to provide information to patients, help resolve patients' concerns and, if necessary, support patients and carers in accessing specialist advocacy services.

Lessons

In this chapter we have described some of the key policy and service developments driving forward collaboration. We have demonstrated some of the educational responses to the collaboration agenda from across the globe and set out a number of innovations around collaborative practice. Whilst in an ideal world the focal point for collaboration is the service user, the reality is that there may be many factors driving collaboration including, for example, service rationalisation and financial calculation. A number of developments at the level of individuals, teams, organisations, sectors and governments have been described and the changing nature of development, as well as the implications for management and accountability of new collaborative practices, discussed.

---

[10] For example, the development of NHS Direct in the UK and Health Link in Alberta, Canada, both of which act as key health information sources for health care users.

New professional profiles are beginning to emerge, reflecting the new models of service provision. It is essential for health and social care professionals that these are viewed as positive, rather than negative developments. Changes in the nature of education and training for health professionals, essential to underpin the developments around collaborative practice and new models of service provision, have also been noted.

Finally, collaboration endorses the development of new relationships with new partners, including an increased recognition of the role of patients and the public in health maintenance. Essentially collaboration embraces the development of a more holistic approach to the provision of health and social services.

Bibliography

Clarence, E. & Painter, C. (1998) Public services under New Labour: collaborative discourses and local networking. *Public Policy and Administration*, **13**(1), 8–22.

Department of Health (1999) *Patient and Public Involvement in the New NHS*. The Stationery Office, London.

Department of Health (2001a) *The Expert Patient: A New Approach to Chronic Disease Management for the Twenty-first Century*. Department of Health, London.

Department of Health (2001b) *Involving Patients and the Public in Health Care: a Discussion Document*. Department of Health, London.

European Observatory on Health Care Systems (2001) *Health Care Systems in Transition – Italy*. WHO Regional Office for Europe, Copenhagen.

Lewin, K. (1946) Action Research and Minority Problems. *Journal of Social Issues*, **2**, 34–6.

Meads, G.D., Chesterman, D., Goosey, D. & Whittington, C. (2003) Practice into theory: learning to facilitate new health and social care partnerships in London. *Learning in Health and Social Care*, **2**(3), 123–36.

Mur, I. & van Raak, A. (2003) Integration of services and the European Union: does EU policy make sense? *International Journal of Integrated Care*, **3**, 1 October.

Niskanen, J. (2002) Finnish care integrated? *International Journal of Integrated Care*, **2**, 1 June.

Scherpbier, A.J.J.A. (Chairman) (2001) *The New Maastricht Curriculum: Best Evidence-Based Medical Education*. Blueprint New Curriculum Committee, University of Maastricht, Maastricht.

Secretary of State for Health (1999) *Saving Lives. Our Healthier Nation*. The Stationery Office, London.

Secretary of State for Health (2000) *The NHS Plan. A Plan for investment. A Plan for Reform*. July. The Stationery Office, London.

Secretary of State for Health (2002) *NHS Reform and Health Care Professions Act*. The Stationery Office, London.

Shaw, S. & Ashcroft, J. (2002) *The Impact of Primary Care Trusts' Emerging Relationships on the Public Health Function*. Department of General Practice and Primary Care, Queen Mary's School of Medicine and Dentistry, London.

Social Exclusion Unit (2001) *National Strategy for Neighbourhood Renewal*. The Stationery Office, London.

The Network: Towards Unity for Health. P. O. Box 616, 6200 MD Maastricht, The Netherlands.

The Network: Towards Unity for Health. Conference, Eldoret, Kenya, 7–11 September 2002.

The Network: Towards Unity for Health. Conference, Australia, 11–15 October 2003.

Wild, A. (2002) *Health Action Zones: Lessons from London.* Report to London Health and Social Care Directorate. University College London, London.

World Health Organization (2000) *World Health Report: Health Systems – Improving Performance.* World Health Organization, Geneva.

Further Reading

Barr, H. (2002) *Interprofessional Education: Today, Yesterday and Tomorrow.* The Learning and Teaching Support Network for Health Sciences & Practice. Occasional Paper No. 1, London.

Centre for the Advancement of Interprofessional Education (CAIPE) (2001) *Bulletin,* **21**.

Department of Environment, Transport and the Regions (1998) *Modern Local Government: In Touch with the People.* The Stationery Office, London.

Department of the Environment, Transport and the Regions (2000) *Joining it up Locally: the Evidence Base. Report of Policy Action Team 17.* The Stationery Office, London.

Grone, O. & Garcia-Barbero, M. (2001) Integrated Care. *International Journal of Integrated Care,* **1**(3), 1 June.

Low, H. & Weinstein, J. (2000) Interprofessional Education. In: *Innovative Education and Training for Care Professionals.* (ed. R. Pierce & J. Weinstein), pp. 205–20. Jessica Kingsley Publishers, London.

Loxley, A. (ed.) (1997) *Collaboration in Health and Welfare: Working with Difference.* Jessica Kingsley Publishers, London.

Meads, G. (2003) Modernising Multi-professional Education. *The Network: Towards Unity for Health Newsletter,* June, **1**, 17–18.

Meads, G., Wild, A., Iwami, M. & Pawlikowska, T. (2004) *International Primary Care in the Twenty-first Century.* University of Warwick, UK.

Robson, C. (1993) *Real World Research* 2nd edn. Blackwell, Oxford.

World Health Organization (1999) *Health 21 – The Health for All Policy Framework for the WHO European Region.* European Health for All Series No. 6. World Health Organization European Regional Office, Copenhagen.

Section III
The Professional Experience

In this section we indicate the individual and collective impact of modern policies based upon collaboration, and detail their historical development, across the world, for different health and social care professions.

Geoffrey Meads and Hugh Barr

7 Personal Learning

Synthesis

It is time to aggregate the learning. This book belongs to a series entitled 'Partnership for Health', the aetiology of which is synthesis. The learning depends not so much on the interprofessional profile of its students or teachers as on making the right connections between its different sections and subjects. In this book these have been internal (to the UK), international (particularly in Chapters one, three and six) and intellectual (or, when employed as advocacy, ideological). Whilst there has been an overarching concern with policy, its impacts and its developmental processes, each of these sections and subjects has been viewed through the prism of multidisciplinary perspectives. To join these perspectives and their subjects together now requires a focus on the individual. What does and will the policy imperative of collaboration actually mean in daily experience for each health and social care professional? What then does it signify for the future of each of their professions?

Our framework for the six relationships of the modern professional helps us to respond to these questions in a suitable summary style which looks to convert aggregate learning into simple messages or a set of syntheses. Under each heading illustrative real life examples are offered. In this chapter the emphasis is mostly on the person. In the next, an authoritative reference document in its own right, the learning is largely about and for corporate entities. Both are equally important. In the past individual practitioners may have often felt, with some justification, that they could ignore political change and set aside management strategies as either remote or irrelevant. The modern professional cannot afford to do so. Health and social care professions are now essentially shaped by their environments and no longer just self directed. Control of one's own destiny, as a professional in a profession, in consequence, depends absolutely upon effective future patterns of external collaboration.

With own profession

The international message is that going solo is no longer an option, even for the super-specialists. Across the world novel forms of national regulation and strategic planning invariably require a collaborative contribution (and dividend) from the individual practitioner and his or her profession. The feminisation of medicine itself, and health care personnel recruitment in general, has paved the way for more collaborative practice within professions. In Albania, South Africa and Bolivia, for example, government directed human resources strategies have created new nursing teams at the frontline of primary care; while parallel approaches in, for example, Austria, Spain and Canada have deliberately created an over supply of doctors to enhance consumer choice, economic export capacity and national government contractual bargaining powers. In the latter the bottom line is a collaborative response by the profession in the style of a trade union on the defensive.

Internally, in the UK, there are multiple modern examples of the new collaborations within professions. Neighbourhood nursing teams, ever extending general medical practice partnerships, oncologists in cancer centres and networks, the surgical squads of Diagnostic and Treatment Centres and geographically sectorised psychiatrists in community mental health services are just some of the most visible examples. Since 1998 the new local contracts for primary care, entitled Primary Medical Services (PMS) have provided a fertile nursery for the growth of new roles and relationships within professions. The following two quotations from recently published PMS evaluations are typical. The first is from a local GP and points to the expansion in the community nursing profession:

'District nurses are increasing their skills in diabetic care and likewise practice nurses are developing their skills in terms of more domiciliary and community based work. We have got a group of nurses to work on nurse triage (as well), which prioritises patients who present to the practice'.

(Riley *et al.* 2003, p. 136)

The second is more succinct and is derived from one of the 12 PMS pilot schemes that in 1999–2000 focused on the needs of people with significant mental health problems. Again, the words are those of a local general practitioner with the subject this time being the overall medical profession: 'Doctors and consultants are sitting down together, working out how they will work...Any (doctor) who is (only) interested in the medical model should be shot!' (Carter *et al.*, 1999, p. 55).

These words point to the open doors and open minds emerging within (and not without a struggle) often previously closed professions in the UK, as elsewhere. If the international message is that going solo is no longer an option then the fundamental idea for the individual professional in his or her daily practice is equally simple: generosity. Professional self interest in response to modernising policies now requires both disciplined expertise and effective generosity. This is the combination which paves the way for the conversion from the (now redundant) self-directed profession to the contemporary 'really managing' health and social care profession[1]. The latter positively interacts with its environment, has

[1] The notion of 'Really Managing Health Care' was developed at City University in the middle 1990s where its Health Management Group was particularly determined to equip clinicians to cope effectively with organisational change and what were regarded as anti-professional political agendas. See Iles (1997) and Iles and Sutherland (2001).

flexible structures, processes and even membership. To survive and succeed takes the ethic and spirit of its past patient encounters into its present and future relationships with one another.

With other professions

The international message is again a simple one. Go interprofessional. Being a health or social care professional now always means accountability 'with' as well as 'for'. Globally, the function and impact of commissioning has become pervasive. No matter whether it be through the not-for-profit but private Kaiser Permanente in California, a mixed status *Entidad Promotora de Salud* (a health promoting enterprise company) in Colombia, or state-run Singhealth in Singapore, commissioning means the pursuit of value for money deals, regardless of individual professional traditions and interests. The drivers of efficiency and effectiveness, increasingly expressed through care management mechanisms and consumerist marketing, mean that professions must collaborate in response. The team, the network and the alliance are the organisational patterns for modern interprofessional relationships.

Internally, in the UK, the original WHO maxim that 'Learning Together *is* Working Together' has been formally adopted not only by New NHS human resource strategies[2] but also at the heart of a comprehensive range of patient-centred policies for integrated (and intermediate) care. The post-1999 National Service Frameworks (NSFs) authorised by the multidisciplinary National Institute for Clinical Excellence and chaired by Sir Michael Rawlins in London are pivotal to the pursuit of integrated care. The *NSF for Older People* provides a classic example of the new policy guidance for interprofessional collaboration. Accordingly, in support of its ministerial aim of 'ensuring fair, high quality, integrated health and social care services for older people' (p. 1) the guidance is:

> 'founded on knowledge-based practice and partnership working between those who... provide services, between different clinicians and practitioners; across different parts of the NHS; the NHS and local government; between the public, voluntary and private sectors'.

(Department of Health, 2001a, p. 4)

Each NSF contains specific targets for implementation and audit. The following sample of the milestones from the Older People's Framework illustrates just how determined the modernisation of relationships across professions can be. For instance this NSF states that by:

---

[2] It often takes, as we have noted elsewhere, at least a decade for the initiatives of international agencies to filter out to national and local orgnaisations. For one example of remarkably similar wording at a distance of 13 years see Department of Health (2001a) and WHO (1988).

'April 2004 NHS primary care trusts will have ensured that: every general practice is using a protocol agreed with local specialist services for the rapid referral and management of those with transient ischaemia attack'.

(p. 16)

and that by April 2003 not only will: 'all general hospitals which care for older people have identified an old age specialist multidisciplinary team with agreed interfaces', but also: 'have completed a skills profile of (all) their staff in relation to the care of older people and have in place education and training programmes to address any gaps identified'.

The Older People's National Service Framework was the fourth such policy guidance to be issued by the post-1997 'New NHS', following NSFs for mental health, coronary heart disease and cancer. It was quickly followed by further Frameworks for diabetes, renal and children services. The emphasis on interprofessional learning and development, epitomised in the last quotation above, is a major feature in each document. It has become the subject of political and, at leadership levels, professional consensus[3]. The College of Occupational Therapists, for example, now declares that it:

'has a strong belief in multi-professional collaboration in terms of pre and post-registration education in order to prepare its members. The College of Occupational Therapy shall respect the needs, practices, unique competencies and responsibilities of other professions.'

(Foreman, 2003)

While even the long established Royal College of Physicians advocates:

'the principle of multi-professional teams working in partnership to deliver health care. It therefore supports the extension for health care professions of the concept of shared learning in the early years of training and multi-professional approaches in care.'

(Foreman, 2002)

This concept is the key idea. Learning together is the essential thrust for cross-professional collaboration. Under the terms of modernising policies it is the profession as much as the environment which is at a formative stage, and which requires educational and explanatory responses. For these to enable individual professions to survive and thrive, such responses will have to be combined and collective.

---

[3] Although associated with the post-1997 Labour Government the initial impetus on shared practice policies came during the last phase of the previous Conservative Government. As the outgoing Secretary of State made clear in his support for an 'evidence-based service' it was considerations of 'cost effectiveness' that were uppermost in his mind in urging professionals and managers to joint 'local strategies to promote clinical effectiveness' (NHS Executive, January 1996, p. 1); while for the leaders of the national nursing and medical professional bodies it was critical that the new clinical effectiveness 'guidelines remain the responsibility of the appropriate professional body (and be) developed at national level', albeit that they 'are produced at local level by teams working in a multidisciplinary way across various sectors of health care'. (NHS Executive, May 1996, pp. 1–4).

With new partners

The above, of course, is not just about the impact on daily practice of interprofessional collaboration. Several of the references include other sectors as well. The declaration by the College of Occupational Therapists, for example, refers not just to collaboration with professions but 'other institutions, statutory and voluntary agencies'; while the NHS Executive's guidance on clinical guidelines drew on a lengthy series of Clinical Effectiveness Bulletins put together through the professions' 'Royal Colleges' partnership with the universities of Leeds and York, a commercial publisher and the Department of Health[4]. Moreover, these references are from the UK, where the NHS is still largely a taxation funded public monopoly. Elsewhere, from Greece to Brazil and Uganda to the Philippines, cross-sectoral collaboration is critical for around half the health and social care resources accessible to professionals.

The international message in relation to new partners is, therefore, that of opportunity spliced by risk. Alternative and additional funds, a new range of employment options, improved facilities and extra therapeutic regimes are all characteristic of modern professional lives in, for example, Canada and Australia, where there is the economic capacity to use private and charitable partnerships to augment an already relatively strong public expenditure base for health and social care. But even in these countries the real risks to professions are apparent. Both remote and not so remote areas now lack medical cover, as doctors (and other professionals) move to the city areas of higher income earning potential. In both countries, as private insurance and supplements have expanded so the proportion of public expenditure has decreased. And elsewhere, in Indonesia and parts of Eastern Europe, for example, full scale privatisation has left health and social care professionals in subordinate staff roles, vertically accountable to non-clinician managers. The very ethical basis for a profession itself, and thence for collaboration by professionals, can very easily fall prey to the competitive market forces unleashed by new partnerships.

It was with the aim of keeping a firm hold on such forces in the UK that the Ministry of Health negotiated its Concordat with leading representatives from across the independent sector (including the major pharmaceutical companies) in 2000–2001. The impact in respect of what policy makers term 'capacity building' for health and social care professionals is dramatic and impressive: national broadband access to the NHS net for clinicians; 500 one stop combined health and social care centres in 2004 and 3000 refurbished primary care team premises by the end of the same year are all dependent on external collaborative ventures. The future list goes on: a countrywide network of privately financed (and sometimes

---

[4] These Bulletins began with Osteoporosis in January 1992, looking to combine professional efforts 'to prevent fractures' and went on to include such other targets as the treatment of depression in primary care, alcohol misuse prevention and the management of subfertility (School of Public Health Consortium 1992–95).

managed) Diagnostic and Treatment Centres, a four-year programme of 29 new hospitals[5], and individual service areas such as learning disability, mental health rehabilitation and community hospitals, where the lead provider role and planning function have now passed on to highly respected and professionally valued voluntary organisations[6].

Such collaborations, as we have discussed in Chapters two, three and five, can have a profound influence on professional performance and accountabilities. For particular individuals and groups they can be disturbing, as well as exciting. For those practising in the UK, therefore, it is as well to learn from those with longer and wider experience of new partnerships. In Indonesia health and social care professions have adopted a traditional legend: 'unity in diversity'. It is the key idea, as powerful in its way as the 'patient-centred' contemporary policies of Western countries. There is a richness in the professional experience from creative collaborations, but they do not change the basic purpose.

With policy actors

Participation in the cyclical process of policy formulation, implementation and evaluation is a global requirement for health and social care professionals. It is so because the global forces outlined in the first section of this book have changed the very nature of policy making itself. Other than in military or authoritarian states – and in these only temporarily – institutional models of the public policy process have been rendered redundant[7]. Universal access to knowledge, modern communications, more comprehensive and higher educational attainment, and extended forms of democratic representation have all played their part in the removal of simple command-and-control structures. Historically these have suited the health if not the social care professions and specialist medical representatives in particular.

The latter have been numbered amongst the relatively few elites with access to and influence in government decisions. Modernisation has changed all that. In many countries, including for example Japan and Portugal, the policies for

---

[5] The new level of collaboration with, in particular, the private sector was prefaced in Chapter 11 of the NHS Plan 2000 (Secretary of State, 2000) and reinforced in successive performance objectives (e.g. Appendix C of Department of Health, 2002).

[6] The 'silent revolution' in English and Welsh community hospitals has seen bed numbers increase while NHS commitments and closures have actually declined, as a result of collaborations by local health and social care professionals with new partners ranging from affluent pop stars to Age Concern (Seamark et al., 2001; Meads, 2001).

[7] For an excellent historic summary and assessment of policy models see John (1998). Institutional models have in the past been seen as favourable to health care professions not simply because leading doctors (and sometimes nurses) have been part of small government-led elites, but also because at each stage and level of the vertical implementation process professional representatives are able to organise themselves effectively to negotiate and effect change. This modification of the institutional model has been known as Incrementalism (Lindblom, 1960).

health and social care are now formally a cross-government departmental function with the Interior Ministry often holding the principal accountability; while
globally alternative forms of decentralisation have wrestled power away from
top-down patriarchs. As a result professionals have to engage with many more
policy players and the notion of strata has given way to 'melting pot' images and,
as we have seen in Chapter three (pp. 40–50) ideas of complex whole systems. The
impact on individual health and social care professions is profound. All of their
members, during the course of their increasingly flexible (and potentially dynamic) careers can expect to occupy, for time limited periods, 'lead' policy
positions for such subjects as governance, audit, external partnerships and even
research. Many find themselves already at the forefront of the organisational
developments emerging from 'modernising policies' whether these be for merged
Sickness Funds in Israel and the Netherlands or centrally determined geographical units for professional human resource distribution, as in Germany and Australia. The institutional model has been replaced already in many countries, and is
now being replaced in others, by a pluralistic model in which the political
administration or civil service can select policy items and approaches from a
wide range of alternative professional (and non-professional) options. Recently
this has been coined by Peter John (1998) the 'Rational Choice' model of policy
making.

   It is a model that has become familiar to most health and social care professionals in the UK, applying, for example, to the development of nurse triage and nurse
practitioner models, the mixed economy of public/private physiotherapy services, pain management procedures, and the multiple progressive extensions in
primary care-led commissioning since the arrival of GP fundholding in 1991. In
the UK environment all inventions are now possible innovations in that every
pilot, zone or exemplar scheme is considered, in policy terms, as fair game for
transfer, adaptation and replication elsewhere. The development of NHS Direct
from its humble origins as a small general practice initiative in Salisbury is,
perhaps, the classic example. As its official policy document proudly declared
in April 2003:

> 'NHS Direct has grown in (just) five years from a small pilot project to a substantial
> national service handling over half a million calls and half a million Internet visitor
> sessions per month. As such it is the world's largest and most successful e-health service
> of its type'.

(Department of Health, 2003, 1:11)

NHS Direct is now a global 'beacon site'. It began simply as the idea of two GPs
and nurses with the support of a local doctoral student and, critically, new
external partners in British Telecom and the Royal College of Nursing[8]. By 2006
it is now expected that the out-of-hours service of every general practice in
England will be integrated with NHS Direct. There could scarcely be a better

---

[8] For origins of this local partnership initiative see Lattimer (1996).

illustration for modern professionals of the significance of being both aware of and active in the policy process.

The key idea, accordingly, has to be that of empowerment. Collaboration in the policy cycle is not an add-on, but a core element in the role of health and social care professionals. It is an opportunity and a responsibility, not a burden or a threat. To see this collaboration this way, for many professions, collectively, and their members, individually, still requires a fundamental attitudinal shift. It is a question of modern but, nevertheless, necessary mindsets.

With public (representatives)

The networks of relationships between the public and the health and social care professions are becoming more numerous and varied as role differentiation impacts equally on both. The public roles now include citizen, consumer, elector, user, advocate, payer, critical friend and, of course, partner. As the relationships increase so do the opportunities for collaboration (and conflict). It is vital to journey together. Exploring modern public-professional relationships should be a shared learning experience.

As Chapter six, especially, has indicated, the new participatory democracies in Latin American countries, where modern health systems are an essential feature often of national regeneration programmes, are at the forefront of international developments. Here, the universal pressures for more direct and personal collaboration by professionals with the public are brought into sharper relief by the problems arising from political instability and poverty. Committed professional involvement with public representatives is crucial to preventive public health, to legitimate priority setting and efficient resource utilisation, to care in the community and to social governance. The particular need depends on the particular context. Not surprisingly, for example, public participation and sound governance go together in war-torn Nicaragua, while in neighbouring and permanently peaceful Costa Rica the strong serious movement in health care is largely associated with preventive public health. In Mexico, local health professions are now incorporated into over 50 000 Community Committees where individual lay persons oversee, for example, educational and audit programmes that combine expert and popular service contributions. Again in Mexico, the nationwide *Opportunidades Sedesol* primary care programme is a construct of three government ministries: responsible for Education, Health and Social Development.

Collaboration between professionals and the public is always a trade off. This is the lesson being learnt in contemporary UK practice. Access to municipal funding under the terms of the 1999 Health Act for NHS professionals is followed by new powers of local authority scrutiny. The control of regulatory and resource allocation bodies such as the Health Professions Council and NHS primary care trusts is achieved in return for an acceptance that the majority on the management boards for each will be lay representatives. Back in Mexico (and Costa Rica) the powerful new local alliances between the public, their representatives and health and social care professionals mean the professional has had to pay a parallel price. In both countries the Government now requires doctors and nurses to undertake at least one year's pre-registration community service in an area of special need, as designated by the Community Committees themselves. It is not too far-fetched to envisage future locally 'owned' NHS Foundation Hospitals operating in a similar mode in England.

Accordingly, the key message is that of negotiation, through power-sharing and shared learning. As professions and the public enter into encounters in increasingly unprecedented and unexpected ways, so the process of health and social care fundamentally changes. In turning to the final professional relationship, with patients (and their proxies) we can see that these changes actually go further. The new collaborations alter what we mean by health itself.

With patient (proxies)

Where Latin America has paved the way for a better appreciation of the changing relationships required individually for health and social care professionals with the public and their representatives, it is to Africa and North America that we should look for the shape of the future, concerning patterns of collaboration with patients, their carers and other proxies. In both continents, in very different circumstances, these patterns are now increasingly those of trade. An exclusive vocational stimulus for professional behaviour is no longer tenable. In both geographical global regions economic pressures have compelled the creation of new creeds of self responsibility for health and social care. In both, as we have described in some detail in relation to the Bamoko Initiative and health maintenance organisations in Chapter three (pp. 38–45), self responsibility and payment go hand in hand. In Africa the aim is to expand and direct demand and resources. In North America it is the opposite: to restrict demand and resources in an overheating health system. In both, the currency of change is the professional encounter with the patient, which has become a transaction. In some of the most commercially developed cities of the world – Hong Kong, London, Singapore, Taiwan and Montreal for example – this has become a shopping experience for patients. Go, for instance, to George Street in central Sydney and within a few hundred metres you can decide which one, or combination, of public/private professional clinics you will 'buy': natural medicine or a GP surgery, a private medical centre or Chinese medicine, a community club's facilities or a holistic health clinic. The collaboration is that of marketing as much as medicine.

In the UK, the trend towards trading professions is less visible but no less marked. The advent of NHS care trusts supplies a simple illustration. Explicitly, with new collaborative organisational ventures between health and social care professionals and their agencies 'for users, carers and patients' the national government guidance asserts that they will demonstrate (author's italics): 'greater potential for *tailored* and integrated care, greater *accessibility* and *one stop shops* for services' (Department of Health, 2001a, p. 3).

Patients are to receive care 'packages' and it is the care trust organisation rather than the profession which 'serves'. In this 'emerging' policy framework the ideas are floated of various proxies for individual patients taking on the 'commissioning' function: local councils, families, carers and even, perhaps, professionals themselves as new 'partners'. But the caveat for such collaborations in this framework is a 'patient-centred' infrastructure of bottom-up accountability quite unlike that which has ever applied to professional conduct and its host organisations before:

> 'Care trusts will need to be accountable to the users of their services and will have representation from Patients' Forums, and the Patients' Advisory and Liaison services, which are being developed, will now apply to Care Trusts. Links with user groups, Citizen's panels etc. will need to be made. In addition, the role of the Local Council's scrutiny committee will be important in the strategic monitoring of Care Trusts.'
>
> (Department of Health, 2001c, p. 6)

England might not yet be Brazil with its National Health Conferences for over 5000 patient delegates[9], but the shift in professional relationships is such that Canning House, the official UK agency for Government supported exchange links with Latin America, has actually begun to host delegations from the likes of Costa Rica and Colombia, eager to explore the British innovations in public and patient participation. Exchange at all levels then, is becoming the central idea in this final area of collaboration.

Lessons

To recapitulate, the sets of syntheses arising from the match between modern policies and practice profoundly affects daily practice and the personal behaviour of each and every health and social care professional. They can do so often in ways that are invisible if not insidious. Our key messages in this chapter have, therefore, been deliberately straightforward. Indicated by international and internal (UK) examples they express the ideas that are framing the new patterns of professional relationships, within and across professions, in the external environment of new policies and partnerships, and with patients and the public.

Going solo is no longer an option; being interprofessional means being a profession; espousing as a partner the legend of 'unity in diversity', empowering oneself through participation in policy developments; negotiating a shared

---

[9] Given its population and market size Brazil is an especially important and influential model for popular collaboration in health and social care, pioneering new co-payment insurance, women's health and municipal funding schemes in its post-1990 Unified Health System (SUS). See Collins *et al.*, (2000).

learning approach in the public interest and trading for real reciprocal patient exchange. These main messages are the sum of personal learning for the collaborative professional experience.

Conclusions

This chapter has focused on the needs of the individual professional. The next is deliberately very different to those that have gone before in substance and in style. It is both a reference and an educational document in its own right. Describing the history and geography of interprofessional education, it ensures that the modern professional experience of collaboration is both properly rounded and grounded.

Bibliography

Carter, Y., Underwood, M., Harding, G., *et al.* (1999) *Personal Medical Services Pilots. Interim Report.* Department of General Practice and Primary Care, Queen Mary and Westfield College, London.

Collins, C., Aravjo, J. & Barbosa, J. (2000) Decentralising the health sector: issues in Brazil. *Health Policy*, **52**, 113–27.

Department of Health (2001a) *National Service Framework for Older People. Executive Summary.* Department of Health, London.

Department of Health (2001c) *Care Trusts. Emerging Framework.* Department of Health, London.

Department of Health (2002) *Improvement, Expansion and Reform. Priorities and Planning Framework* 2003–2006. Department of Health, London.

Department of Health (2003) *Developing NHS Direct.* Department of Health, Leeds.

Foreman, D. (2002) The management of shared learning between health care professions. *International Journal of Allied Human Resource Management*, **3**(3), 147–62.

Foreman, D. (2003) Working together for individual health. Inaugural Lecture, University of Derby, UK.

Iles, V. (1997) *Really Managing Health Care.* Open University Press, Buckingham.

Iles, V. & Sutherland, K. (2001) *Organisational Change.* National Coordinating Centre for Service Delivery and Organisation, London School of Hygiene and Tropical Medicine, London.

John, P. (1998) *Analysing Public Policy.* Continuum, London.

Lattimer, V., Smith, H., Hungin, P., Gasper, A. & George, S. (1996) Future provision of out-of-hours primary medical care: a survey with two general practitioner networks. *British Medical Journal*, **312**, 352–6.

Lindblom, C. (1960) The science of muddling through. *Public Administration Review*, **38**, 79–88.

Meads, G. (2001) Rediscovering community hospitals. *British Journal of General Practice*, **51**, 91–2.

NHS Executive (January 1996) *Promoting Clinical Effectiveness.* Department of Health, Leeds.

NHS Executive (May 1996) *Clinical Guidelines*. Department of Health, Leeds.

Riley, A., Harding, G., Meads, G., Underwood, M. & Carter, Y. (2003) An evaluation of personal medical services: the times they are a-changin'. *Journal of Interprofessional Care*, 17(2), 127–39.

School of Public Health Consortium (1992–1995) *Effective Health Care Bulletins*. University of Leeds, UK.

Secretary of State for Health (1999) *Saving Lives. Our Healthier Nation*. The Stationery Office, London.

Secretary of State for Health (2000) *The NHS Plan. A Plan for Investment. A Plan for Reform*. The Stationery Office, London.

Seamark, D., Moore, B., Tucker, H. & Seamark, K. (2001) Community hospitals for the new millennium. *British Journal of General Practice*, **51**, 125–7.

WHO, African Regional Committee (1988) Document AFR/RC37/R1. BamokoInitiative, Mali.

Further Reading

Department of Health (2001b) *Working Together, Learning Together: a Framework for Lifelong Learning in the NHS*. Department of Health, London.

WHO Study Group on Multi-professional Education (1998) *Learning to Work Together for Health: the Team Approach*. World Health Organization Technical Report Series No. 769, Geneva.

8 Learning Together

Purpose

Learning about collaboration is one thing: learning how to collaborate is quite another. It is active – interactive between the parties who need to collaborate. It happens during education and practice: interprofessional education where professions learn with, from and about each other to forge effective working relations, interprofessional practice where those relationships are tested and developed. Interprofessional working is the axis around which collaboration within and between organisations and with patients, carers and communities revolves.

This chapter reviews the development of interprofessional education worldwide from a corporate perspective during the past 30 years.[1] It leads into two further books in preparation for this series, one establishing the evidence base for interprofessional education (Barr *et al.*, 2005) and the other offering practical advice about developing, delivering and evaluating interprofessional education programmes (Freeth *et al.*, 2005).

The World Health Organization

The origin of interprofessional education is widely attributed to a seminal report from an expert group convened by the Geneva headquarters of the World Health Organization (WHO, 1987a). That report, *Learning Together to Work Together for Health*, did much to inspire interprofessional education initiatives around the world and remains the most authoritative statement. Its significance, however, lay in reaffirming and reinforcing much that the WHO had said before while collating and presenting prior experience to further WHO objectives. Its support for interprofessional education sprang from its mounting concern about the relevance of health professions' education, especially medical education, over many years, as Tope (1996) has assiduously documented. In 1973, an expert committee reviewing medical education had seen interprofessional and

---

[1] It is based on a longer review of the development of interprofessional education worldwide, by Hugh Barr, which is periodically updated, to be found on www.caipe.org.uk

traditional programmes as complementary. Its members believed that interprofessional education would improve job satisfaction, increase public appreciation of the health care team and encourage a holistic response to patients' needs. Each member state in the WHO was charged with the task of providing interprofessional programmes, beginning with demonstration projects (WHO, 1973). By the time delegates met in Alma Ata (WHO, 1978), interprofessional education was already firmly included in the emerging WHO strategy to promote 'Health for All by the year 2000'.

The 1987 WHO group was convinced that community oriented, interprofessional education of health personnel had an important place in strategies for achieving Health for All which the WHO had set out a decade before (WHO, 1978). Its conviction was confirmed by examples quoted of interprofessional education in no fewer than 14 countries: Algeria, Australia, Canada, Egypt, France, Israel, Mexico, Nepal, Pakistan, the Philippines, the Sudan, Sweden, the UK and the USA.

Nor was the WHO the only international body involved. The Organisation for Economic Cooperation and Development had convened a conference in 1977 to foster exchange of experience between interprofessional education programmes in different countries. It gave examples of core curricula designed to develop the 'Regional University' to unite schools for the health professions in a common mission in response to the needs of the societies they served (OECD, 1977).

The first acknowledgement of interprofessional education by the World Federation of Medical Education came in 1988 (WFME, 1988). In the following year it called upon all nations globally to train their doctors in close association with the training provided for the other health professions, a message that it reinforced in 1993 (WFME, 1994). The ethos of teamwork was established, said Lord Walton (then President of the WFME), through interprofessional education. The outcome would be more cost-effective doctors, better equipped to work as members of health teams for the benefit of both patients and communities (Walton, 1995).

The degree to which the WHO and other world organisations influenced national developments differed from country to country. Reference to the WHO is conspicuous by its absence from USA and found only occasionally in UK sources, but more often in those from smaller European states and developing countries.

Europe

Building upon the seminal report from its headquarters in Geneva, the WHO Regional Office for Europe convened a workshop in Copenhagen which further advanced the case for interprofessional education. Participants believed that such education would help health professions' students with complementary roles in teams as they came to appreciate the value of working together, by defining and solving problems within a common frame of reference. Participatory learning methods would facilitate modification of reciprocal attitudes, foster team spirit, identify and value respective roles, whilst effecting change in both practice and the professions. All this would support the development of integrated health care, based upon common attitudes, knowledge and skills. Programmes were to be mounted collaboratively at every educational level and evaluated systematically (d'Ivernois & Vodoratski, 1988).

Two reviews of interprofessional education in Europe have been conducted. The first informed discussions during the WHO workshop (d'Ivernois *et al.*, 1988). The second, commissioned by the Council of Europe (European Health Committee, 1993), tracked subsequent developments. Both focused upon programmes in particular universities rather than the workplace, with little reference to the context in which they had been instigated.

The review for the WHO included reports on developments in Belgium (Piette, 1988), Finland (Isokoski, 1988), France (d'Ivernois *et al.*, 1988), Greece (Lanara, 1988), Portugal (Rendas, 1988), Sweden (Areskog, 1988a), the UK (Clarke, 1988; Thomson, 1988), the USSR (Shigan, 1988) and Yugoslavia (Kovacic, 1988). Those in France and Sweden attracted most interest subsequently in other countries.

The second review for the Council of Europe took the form of a questionnaire to all its member states, with follow-up visits to some. Information was received from Cyprus, Germany, Holland, Liechtenstein, Luxembourg, Norway, Spain, Switzerland and Turkey. In addition, working party members were able to report developments in their home states, namely Austria, Belgium, Czechoslovakia, Denmark, Finland, France, Hungary, Portugal, Sweden and the UK. Findings were, however, disappointing. Interprofessional education had reportedly been implemented in only a few European centres. Postgraduate developments were, said the report, spread thinly. In most countries they took the form of 'on the job' short courses, joint learning leading to diplomas or degrees being the exception. Most developments were in response to local initiatives. None of the member states reportedly having national policies to encourage interprofessional education. Except in The Netherlands, central government departments of health and education were, according to the report, unaware of what was taking place in their own countries. The Council of Europe endorsed the report and outlined a four-stage strategy to promote interprofessional education in its member states. These were the dissemination of information through seminars, access to consultants to help in planning programmes, implementation of those programmes and systematic evaluation before and before the intervention (European Health Committee, 1993; see also Barr 1994a and Jones, 1994).

A European Network for the Development of Multi-Professional Education in Health Sciences (EMPE) was established in 1987 (Goble, 1994a, b), and continued until 2000, when it merged with the Network for Community-Based Medical Education (as it was then known) (see below). Its newsletter and annual conference during the intervening years provided opportunities to exchange experience between educational institutions mounting 'multi-professional' courses throughout Europe.

Interprofessional education developed in the UK on a larger scale than in most other European states. Why this has been so is not obvious except in more recent years. The first UK initiatives were reported in the 1960s and 1970s. Many promoted team development in primary and community care. Most were brief, work-based and short-lived. Few were recorded. Reports of national conferences convened jointly by professional associations and regulatory bodies did, however, capture the essence of these pioneering developments (England, 1979; Thwaites, 1993; Loxley, 1997). Credit for translating local initiatives into a nationwide movement went to the Health Education Authority, which engaged representatives of primary care teams in a rolling programme of workshops designed to implement health promotion strategies (Spratley 1990a, b). Meanwhile, a succession of high profile reports from inquiries into cases of abuse prompted joint training in child protection.

Interprofessional education was also taking root in universities. Exeter was first in the field in 1973, when it launched continuing education programmes shared between health and social care professions, followed in 1986 by the first joint masters course (Pereira Gray *et al.*, 1993). Other masters courses followed (Leathard, 1992; Storrie, 1992).

Despite conventional wisdom to the effect that interprofessional education should wait until students had qualified, undergraduate initiatives also attracted passing mention during the 1970s (Mortimer, 1979). The first to be more fully reported was at Salford, which drew on experience from Adelaide, Australia, and Linkoping, Sweden, to develop problem-based learning (PBL) as a means to cultivate collaboration between professions (Davidson & Lucas, 1995).

The Conservative Governments of Margaret Thatcher and John Major between 1979 and 1997 put their faith in the virtues of competitive markets, which seemed at first to undermine much hard work to introduce collaboration. They continued, however, to espouse collaboration to implement health and social care reforms backed by calls for 'shared learning' and 'joint training' (Barr, 1994b; Leathard, 1994; Mackay *et al.*, 1995; Loxley, 1997) without apparent sense of contradiction.

Commitment to collaboration was renewed and reinforced following the election of the Labour Government in 1997. While competitive undercurrents remained, the emphasis was now upon integration, partnership and joined-up thinking, from grass-roots practice through to the corridors of Whitehall. Collaboration, as Chapter two argued, has been as much between organisations, and with patients, carers and communities, as between practising professionals.

No longer on the margins, interprofessional education was to be built into the mainstream of professional education across health and social care to promote such collaboration. No longer mostly after qualification, elements of 'common learning' were required in all undergraduate programmes for all the health and social care professions. Interprofessional education itself would be developed and managed in partnership between employers and universities.

Interprofessional education has become more an instrument to effect change than a vehicle through which to improve understanding based upon mutual respect between professions. This has destabilised roles and generated new found stress between professions, as boundaries have become permeable, posing even greater changes for interprofessional education. Earlier models of interprofessional education were rendered less than adequate. Engendering trust and understanding between professions, however, remained the precondition to ensure concerted commitment to change in furtherance of the Government's modernisation agenda (Secretary of State for Health, 1997).

CAIPE was founded in 1987, following the first flush of interprofessional developments. Caught, by then, in a more competitive and less sympathetic environment, it held fast to the convictions of its founders about the efficacy of interprofessional education in improving teamwork and, in turn, the quality of care. Its self-appointed remit was to promote interprofessional education as a means to improve collaboration between practitioners in health and social care, working with and through its members to provide a network for information exchange and discussion by means of conferences and seminars, a bulletin, occasional papers, periodic surveys and reviews. That brief changed as collaboration gained ascendancy over competition, following the change of Government in 1997, when interprofessional education began to enjoy official backing. No longer championing an unpopular cause, CAIPE was working with the grain. Its task, now, was to inform the new wave of developments, drawing upon but going beyond lessons learned from past experience as the situation demanded, challenging ill-conceived innovations while increasingly recognising the need to secure the evidence base for interprofessional education (see www.caipe.org.uk).

Other central bodies also supported developments in interprofessional education as it moved into the mainstream of higher and professional education. The three Learning and Teaching Support Networks for the health and social care professions joined forces to support developments in universities and to provide a clearing house through its website (www.triple-ltsn.kcl.ac.uk). The Association for the Study of Medical Education drew other professions into its debates through interprofessional conferences (www.asme.org.uk). The Learning for Partnership Network, under the wing of CAIPE, facilitated exchange on interprofessional matters centrally between regulatory and professional bodies.

A survey commissioned by CAIPE towards the end of the 1980s found 695 examples of interprofessional education in Great Britain. Most were short and formed part of continuing professional development (Shakespeare *et al.*, 1989, as summarised by Horder, 1995). A follow-up survey for the whole of the UK found 455 initiatives, but based upon a much lower response rate which belied the increasing prevalence of interprofessional education in the intervening years (Barr & Waterton, 1996). The number of interprofessional education programmes since then has increased markedly, so much so that further surveys have been precluded on grounds of cost. Tracking fast-changing developments has become ever more problematic, rendering findings soon out of date. Furthermore, interprofessional education increasingly comprises strands woven into the fabric of professional education, making it harder to identify and quantify.

The other main concentration of interprofessional education in Europe is in the Nordic countries, notably Sweden, Norway and Finland. Of developments in

Sweden, undergraduate interprofessional education at the regional health university at Linkoping attracted most interest and came to be regarded as a classic study worldwide. Capitalising upon the amalgamation of schools for medicine, nursing, occupational and physical therapy, laboratory assistants and social assistants, Linkoping introduced a common ten-week programme for all its undergraduate students at the start of their first year to cultivate collaboration. Common curricula employed problem-based learning methods (Areskog, 1988a, b, 1992, 1994, 1995; Davidson & Lucas, 1995). Other developments in Sweden have been reported at the University of Goteborg, which had postgraduate programmes in public health; Vanersborg University College, which had an undergraduate programme in European Health Sciences (Freden, 1997); and in Stockholm in association with the Karolinska Institute, through a number of interprofessional training wards.

The Norwegian Government decided that undergraduate interprofessional education should be piloted in Tromso, between students of medicine in the University and of other professions in the College of Health (Ekeli, 1996). While there were similarities between developments in Linkoping and Tromso, the latter included a wider range of health professions, ran shared studies concurrently with uni-professional studies and focused less exclusively upon problem-based learning (Freden, 1997).

The first reported interprofessional education programmes in Finland were in health administration at the universities of Tampere (Isokoski, 1988) and Kuopio (d'Ivernois et al., 1988). These pioneers were followed by a number of programmes further north in Oulu Polytechnic, which applied a model of holistic care (Lamsa et al., 1994), while staff from the University of Oulu Medical School introduced an innovative programme in family systems education, employing a bio-psychosocial model (Larivaara & Taanila, 2004).

The Nordic Network for Interprofessional Education (NIPNET) was established in 2000. It facilitates mutual support and stimulus by email correspondence and an annual conference for interprofessional activists starting with Finland, Norway and Sweden but seeking to extend to include Denmark, Iceland, the Baltic States and adjoining parts of Russia (see www.nipnet.org).

Interprofessional education programmes throughout the remainder of Europe have been widely scattered. Noteworthy amongst them was the Medical Faculty of the University Paris-Nord, at Bobigny in France, which introduced a common core of studies in nursing, biology, health administration and clinical psychology for first year undergraduates from 1984 onwards, followed by interprofessional masters courses (d'Ivernois et al., 1988).

North America

Direct reference to the role of the WHO in promoting interprofessional education is conspicuously lacking in the North American literature, where foundations were being laid as early as the 1930s with the shift from learning by rote to problem solving (Dewey, 1939). Later, during the 1960s and 1970s, the new systems approach gained, according to Kuehn (1998), widespread popularity as a framework that could support the more interactive and changing environment of health care education and delivery. At the same time, broader-based movements in higher education toward interdisciplinary interaction were prompting the re-examination of health professional education from an interdisciplinary perspective. This, Kuehn reminds us, was also the time when Piaget (1970) was calling for a more collaborative approach in both teaching and research. It was the time, too, when the 1971 Rockefeller Foundation Task Force on Higher Education called for changes in professional education to obviate 'the stifling effects of rigid curricula that inhibited any movement towards interactive or creative endeavours' (Newman, 1971). A year later, the Carnegie Commission had proposed a lessening of emphasis upon professional boundaries, a holistic approach and the building of curricular bridges to combat the inherent parochialism of professional education. But perhaps the most powerful moves towards collaborative education, thought Kuehn, had come in the 1990s with the rush to control the economics of both health care and health professions education with the advent of health maintenance organisations and managed care (see Chapter two).

The first published reports about interprofessional education in North America appeared during the 1960s (Lewis & Resnick, 1966; Kenneth, 1969; Szasz, 1969). Some were associated with the introduction of teamwork in primary care (Beckard, 1974; Fry et al., 1974). As far back as 1958, Silver, in his description of teamwork in general practice, had noted the opportunity for informal learning between team members occasioned by the ease of communication (Silver, 1958).

Pioneering interprofessional programmes reported by Baldwin (1996) in North American universities included British Columbia, Nevada, Hawaii and Sherbrooke. During the 1970s six medical schools, Nevada, Michigan State, North Carolina, Washington, Utah and California at San Francisco, devised a common model for team training. Developments differed in emphasis. Some, like British Columbia and Minnesota, had a more academic focus; others, like Miami, Colorado and Indiana, a more clinical focus; yet others, like Kentucky, a community focus, while Nevada and Georgia sought to strike a balance. These university-based initiatives were complemented by work-based initiatives, support for 'interdisciplinary training' being noteworthy from the Veterans Administration in the context of interdisciplinary care teams, which generated a cadre of team trainers nationally, for the care of the elderly and other client groups.

Many of the early developments enjoyed federal support, much of which had been withdrawn by 1980, although some continued from the Bureau of Health Professions of the Health Resources and Services Administration. Philanthropic foundations played an increasingly major part. The Pew Charitable Trust Foundation published a report strongly advocating interdisciplinary training for future health professionals (O'Neil, 1993). The Hartford Foundation provided grants, for example, for the Geriatric Interdisciplinary Team Training Program (GITT) (Siegler et al., 1998), while the W.K. Kellogg Foundation funded university-community partnerships and the Robert Wood Johnson Foundation funded the Partnership for Quality Education Initiative to support the development of nurse practitioner/physician teams in primary care.

The Community/Campus Partnerships for Health movement gathered momentum later, linking programmes in the USA and other countries to cultivate collaboration between universities and neighbourhoods to provide health services and thereby to develop practice-based community-oriented curricula (Foley & Feletti, 1993; Seifer & Maurana, 1998). These developments were closely linked with the service learning movement associated with the Health Professions Schools in Service to the Nation Program (HPSISNP), which examined the impact of such learning on students, faculties and communities (Gelmon et al., 1998). Similar partnerships have also been established that reach beyond health care. These adopt a community development model and involve as wide as possible a range of academic disciplines and practice professions in response to needs identified in consultation with local communities.

Interprofessional education in North America comprises interlocking networks for communication and shared learning with many new initiatives underway, supported by both Government and foundation moneys. One of the longest established is the Annual Interdisciplinary Health Care Team Conference that brings together teachers and trainers who employ interprofessional education to promote teamwork in hospital and community settings. At the time of writing, this Conference was taking the lead in engaging like-minded North American organisations in discussions designed to cultivate closer collaboration at national and international level leading to proposals for an International Association for the Study of Interprofessional Education provisionally based in Vancouver, Canada.

Australasia

In Australia plans were made during the 1970s for interprofessional education in ten medical schools, although only one got off the ground. This was at the University of Adelaide, in collaboration with the South Australia Institute of Technology, where federal funding made it possible to mount joint programmes for 600 undergraduates on community health and practice. Federal funding was withdrawn towards the end of the 1980s, but the programme not only continued but was also extended to include other institutions, bringing in students from a wider range of professions. Shared undergraduate studies ceased in 1992 for lack of resources, although shared postgraduate studies continued, as did practice workshops (Piggot, 1980; Davidson & Lucas, 1995; Vanclay, 1995; Tope 1996; Graham & Wealthall, 1999). Plans for similar developments were reportedly getting underway at the University of Newcastle during the early 1990s, where the focus became the development of flexible, need oriented, 'knowledge-able' health and social care professionals (personal communication with M. McMillan, University of Newcastle, Australia, 2003). In addition, a WHO Regional Training

Centre in the College of Medicine at the University of New South Wales had been running advanced and postgraduate courses for some years for a range of health personnel from Asian and Pacific countries (Vanclay, 1995).

Graham and Wealthall (1999) reported that a number of other Australian universities, including Curtin, La Trobe, South Australia, Sydney and Queensland, had adopted some form of common curriculum. They nevertheless observed that 'the exigencies of university life' in Australia inhibited the flexibility required to foster such developments, although stakes were less high for continuing professional development. Moves were, however, afoot to increase interprofessional learning experiences for all professional groups.

Significantly, the Australian and New Zealand Association for Medical Education (ANZAME), widened its membership to include all health professions, established a special interest section on 'multi-professional education' and launched a 'multidisciplinary' journal (see www.anzame.unsw.edu.au).

Developing countries

As well as those referred to in Chapter six interprofessional education has been reported in several developing countries: Algeria, the Cameroons, the Dominican Republic (Vinal, 1987; Kuehn, 1998), Fiji, the Philippines, Thailand (WHO, 1987b; Tope, 1996), the Sudan (Hamad, 1982; Tope, 1996), Lebanon (Makaram, 1995), Colombia (Penuela, 1999) and South Africa (Lazarus et al., 1998). While some of these initiatives are similar in form and composition to those reported in developed countries, others extend the range of professions to include, for example, agriculturists, engineers and sanitarians engaged in public health and community development projects. Some are also designed to create a flexible workforce that the country can afford, unfettered by narrow definitions of professionalism and preconceived demarcations inherited from colonial powers.

Bajaj (1994), for example, described a competency-based approach to interprofessional education in India and its inclusion at all stages in the educational continuum from pre-qualifying programmes through orientation to beginning practice and to continuing education. This was built around a core curriculum combined with problem-based learning to acquire and demonstrate competence in teamwork. Interprofessional education, said Bajaj, had to address the particular health problems of the community and therefore be community-based. Predetermined institutional frameworks had to be replaced or enlarged. Village schoolteachers, for example, had been helped to develop their role in primary health care by participating in shared learning with other health personnel.

Having invested heavily in interprofessional education in the USA, the W.K. Kellogg Foundation backed initiatives in developing countries through its TUFH Program. This comprised 20 projects in 11 countries in Latin America and the Caribbean to integrate the university, the services and the community and foster interprofessional collaboration (Richards, 1993; UNI, 1999; Goble, 2003) and in South Africa (Lazarus et al., 1998).

Community-oriented education for health sciences

Two international movements grew out of the lead given by the WHO, with which others have become associated over the years. The more cohesive is 'The Network' based in Maastricht in The Netherlands, established in 1979 to promote community-based medical education by means of problem-based learning. It enjoys official relations with the UN and the WHO, and has some 300 member institutions worldwide as Chapter six reports. The Network has become increasingly interested in, and committed to, interprofessional education following mergers with the European Network for the Development of Multi-professional Education (EMPE) and, more recently, WHO Towards Unity for Health, and joint activities with Community-Campus Partnership (see www.the-networktufh.org).

The other movement loosely links groups like the US Interdisciplinary Health Teams Conference, CAIPE, NIPNET with like-minded individuals and programmes worldwide. The *Journal of Interprofessional Care* is its vehicle to exchange experience and extend mutual support. Unlike The Network, this movement has the promotion of interprofessional education and practice as its primary goal; involves health and social care as equal partners; and explores wider-ranging models and learning methods in interprofessional education.

These two movements nevertheless have much in common, both echoing the WHO clarion call, and both acting on the belief that education, including interprofessional education, has the power to effect change in response to the expressed needs of patients and communities as partners.

Learning between developed and developing countries

Systematic comparison between interprofessional education programmes internationally is overdue. Similarities are striking between developed countries in Australasia, Europe and North America, despite limited opportunities, until recently, to exchange ideas and experience. Differences between the so-called developed and developing world are more marked. While developed countries have concentrated on preparation for practice with individuals and families, developing countries have grasped the significance of interprofessional education and practice to mobilise resources for community development and public works. Sources assembled in this chapter challenge any assumptions that Europe was the cradle of interprofessional education from which it has reached out to developing countries (Goble, 2003). The thread of corporate commitment runs rather between the USA and Latin America and beyond, leaving Europe in relative isolation, save for a handful of dedicated interprofessional exponents committed to work with and through international institutions. Above all, sources reviewed in this chapter, and Chapter three, point to the need for more dialogue, exchange and mutual support between developed and developing countries so that each can learn from the distinctive experience of the other in the best tradition of interprofessional education.

Bibliography

Areskog, N-H. (1988a) Multi-professional team training within the health care sector in Sweden. In: *Multi-professional Education of Health Personnel in the European Region*. (eds J-F. Ivernois & V. Vodoratski.) Annex 7. World Health Organization, Copenhagen.

Areskog, N-H. (1988b) The need for multi-professional health education in undergraduate studies. *Medical Education*, **22**, 251–2.

Areskog, N-H. (1992) The New Medical Education at the Faculty of Health Sciences, Linkoping University – a challenge for both students and teachers. *Scandinavian Journal of Medical Education*, **2**, 1–4.

Areskog, N-H. (1994) Multi-professional education at the undergraduate level – the Linkoping Model. *Journal of Interprofessional Care*, **8**(3), 279–82.

Areskog, N-H. (1995) Multi-professional education at the undergraduate level. In: *Interprofessional Relations in Health Care* (eds K. Soothill, L. Mackay & C. Webb), Edward Arnold, London, pp. 125–39.

Bajaj, J. (1994) Multi-professional education as an essential component of effective health service. *Medical Education*, **28**, (Supplement 1).

Baldwin, D. (1996) Some historical notes on interdisciplinary and interprofessional education and practice in health care in the USA. *Journal of Interprofessional Care*, **10**(2), 173–88.

Barr, H. (1994a) Multi-professional education in Europe: a European Health Committee Report. *Journal of Interprofessional Care*, **8**(1), 116.

Barr, H. (1994b) *Perspectives on Shared Learning*. CAIPE, London.

Barr, H. & Waterton, S. (1996) *Interprofessional Education in Health and Social Care: the Report of a United Kingdom Survey*. CAIPE, London.

Barr, H., Koppel, I., Reeves, S., Freeth, D. & Hammick, M. (2005) *Effective Interprofessional Education: Argument, Assumption and Evidence*. Blackwell Science, Oxford.

Beckard, R. (1974) Organisational issues in the team delivery of comprehensive health care. *Milbank Memorial Fund Quarterly*, **50**, 287–316.

Clarke, W.D. (1988) The British Life Assurance Trust Centre for Health and Medical Education (BLAT) and Multi-professional Training. In: *Multi-professional Education for Health Personnel in the European Region*. (eds J-F. d'Ivernois & V. Vodoratski) Annex 8. WHO, Copenhagen.

Davidson, L. & Lucas, J. (1995) Multi-professional education in the undergraduate health professions curriculum: observations from Adelaide, Linkoping and Salford. *Journal of Interprofessional Care*, **9**(2), 163–76.

Dewey, J. (1939) Experience and education. In: *Selected Readings on Philosophy and Adult Education*. (ed. S. B. Merriam, 1984) Robert E. Krieger Publishing Company, Malabar, Florida.

Ekeli, B-V. (1996) *Multi-professional health care education in Tromso*. In: *Introduction to Holistic Care*. (eds A. Lamsa & M. Paatalo) pp. 74–5. Oulu Polytechnic School of Health, Oulu, Finland.

England, H. (ed.) (1979) *Education for Cooperation in Health and Social Work: Papers from the Symposium in Interprofessional Learning*, University of Nottingham, July 1979. Royal College of General Practitioners, London.

European Health Committee (1993) *Multi-professional Education for Health Personnel*. Council of Europe, Strasbourg.

Foley, H. & Felleti, G. (1993) The Hawaii Education Community Partnership Programme. *Annals of Community-Oriented Education*, **6**, 125–40.

Freden, L. (1997) Unpublished presentation to the London conference entitled 'All Together Better Health'.

Freeth, D., Hammick, M., Barr, H., Koppel, I. & Reeves, S. (2005) *Effective Interprofessional Education: Development, Delivery and Evaluation*. Blackwell Science, Oxford.

Fry, R., Lech, B. & Rubin, I. (1974) Working with the primary care team; the first intervention. In: *Making Health Care Teams Work*. (eds H. Wise *et al.*) pp. 27–59. Ballinger, Cambridge, Mass.

Gelmon, S., Holland, B., Shinnamon, A. & Morris, B. (1998) Community-based education and services: the HPSISN experience. *Journal of Interprofessional Care*, **12**(3), 257–72.

Goble, R. (1994a) Multi-professional education in Europe: an overview. In: *Going Interprofessional: Working Together for Health and Welfare*. (ed. A. Leathard). pp. 175–87 Routledge, London.

Goble, R. (1994b) Multi-professional education: European Network for Development of Multi-professional Education in Health Sciences (EMPE). *Journal of Interprofessional Care*, **8**(1), 85–92.

Goble, R. (2003) Multi-professional education: global perspectives. In: *Interprofessional Collaboration: from Policy to Practice in Health and Social Care*. (ed. A. Leathard) pp. 324–34. Brunner-Routledge, Hove.

Graham, J. & Wealthall, S. (1999) Interdisciplinary education for health professions: taking the risk for community gain. *Focus on Health Professional Education: a Multidisciplinary Journal*, **1**(1), 49–69.

Hamad, B. (1982) Interdisciplinary field training research and rural development programme. *Medical Education*, **16**, 105–7.

Horder, J. (1995) Interprofessional education for primary health and community care; present and future needs. In: *Interprofessional Relations in Health Care*. (eds K. Soothill, L. Mackay & C. Webb) pp. 140–62. Edward Arnold, London.

Isokoski, M. (1988) Multi-professional training for primary health care administration: The Finnish experience. In: *Multi-professional Education for Health Personnel in the European Region*. (eds J-F. d'Ivernois & V. Vodoratski). Annex 3. World Health Organization, Copenhagen.

d'Ivernois, J-F. & Vodoratski, V. (1988) *Multi-professional Education for Health Personnel in the European Region*. World Health Organization, Copenhagen.

d'Ivernois, J-F. Cornillot, P. & Zomer, Y. (1988) Experiences of multi-professional education at the Medical Faculty of University Paris-Nord, Bobigny. In: *Multi-professional Education for Health Personnel in the European Region*. (eds J-F. d'Ivernois & V. Vodoratski). Annex 4. World Health Organization, Copenhagen.

Jones. R.V. (1994) Multi-professional education in Europe: a European Health Committee Report. *Journal of Interprofessional Care*, **8**(1), 115–6.

Kenneth, H. (1969) Medical and nursing students learn together. *Nursing Outlook*, **17** (11), 46–9.

Kuehn, A.F. (1998) Collaborative health professional education: an interdisciplinary mandate for the third millennium. In: *Collaboration: a Health Care Imperative*. (ed. T.J. Sullivan). pp. 419–65. McGraw-Hill, New York.

Lamsa, A., Hietanen, I. & Lamsa, J. (1994) Education for holistic care: a pilot programme in Finland. *Journal of Interprofessional Care*, **8**(1), 31–44.

Larivaara, P. & Taanila, A. (2004) Towards interdisciplinary Family-Oriented Teams in primary care: evaluation of a training programme. *Journal of Interprofessional Care*, **18**(2), 153–64.

Lazarus, J., Meservey, P. M., Joubert, R., Lawrence, G., Ngobeni, F. & September, V. (1998) The South African Community Partnerships: towards a model for interdisciplinary health personnel education. *Journal of Interprofessional Care*, **12**(13), 279–88.

Leathard, A. (1992) Interprofessional Education at South Bank Polytechnic. *Journal of Interprofessional Care*, **6**(1), 17–24.

Leathard, A. (1994) *Going Interprofessional: Working Together for Health and Welfare*. Routledge, London.

Lewis, C. & Resnick. B. (1966) Relative orientation of students of medicine and nursing to ambulatory patient care. *Journal of Medical Education*, **41**, 162–6.

Loxley, A. (1997) *Collaboration in Health and Welfare: Working with Difference*. Jessica Kingsley Publishers, London.

Mackay, L., Soothill, K. & Webb, C. (1995) Troubled times: the context for interprofessional collaboration? In: *Interprofessional Relations in Health Care*. (eds K. Soothill, L. Mackay & C. Webb). Edward Arnold, London.

Mortimer, E. (1979) Interdisciplinary learning at the qualifying and post-qualifying stages. In: *Education for Cooperation in Health and Social Work: Papers from the Symposium in Interprofessional Learning*. (ed. H. England) University of Nottingham, July 1979. Royal College of General Practitioners, London, cited in England (1979).

Newman, F. (1971) (ed.) *Report on Higher Education*. US Government Printing Office, Washington DC.

O'Neil, E. (1993) *Health Professions Education for the Future. Schools in Service to the Nation*. Pew Health Professions Commission. Pew Charitable Trust Foundation, San Francisco.

Organisation for Economic and Cultural Development. (1977) *Health, Higher Education and the Community – Towards a Regional Health University*. Report of an International Conference. Centre for Educational Research and Innovation, Paris.

Penuela, M. (1999) The use of interdisciplinary/multi-professional education within a community-based curriculum at the Universidad del Norte of Barranquilla, Colombia. *Newsletter of the Network of Community-Oriented Educational Institutions for Health Sciences*. Number 30.

Pereira Gray, D., Goble, R., Openshaw, S. *et al.* (1993) Multi-professional education at the Postgraduate Medical School, University of Exeter. *Annals of Community-Oriented Education*, **6**, 181–90.

Piaget, J. (1970) The epistemology of interdisciplinary relationships. In: *Interdisciplinarity: Problems of Teaching and Research in Universities*. (ed. L. Apostel), pp. 127–39. Organisation of Economic Cooperation and Development, Nice.

Piette, D. (1986) Multi-professional training in health education: the project of the Inter-university Group for the French-speaking area of Belgium. In: *Multi-professional Education for Health Personnel in the European Region*. (eds J-F. d'Ivernois & V. Vodoratski). Annex 2. World Health Organization, Copenhagen.

Richards, R.W. (1993) Community Partnership: redirecting health professions education towards primary health care. *Annals of Community-Oriented Education*, 6, 219–30.

Secretary of State for Health (1997) *The New NHS: Modern, Dependable*. Department of Health, London.

Seifer, S. & Maurana, C. (1998) Editorial. *Journal of Interprofessional Care*, 12, 3. 253–4.

Shakespeare, H., Tucker, W. & Northover, J. (1989) *Report of a National Survey of Interprofessional Education in Primary Care*. CAIPE, London.

Siegler, E.L., Hyer, K., Fulmer, T. & Mezey, M. (1998) *Geriatric Interdisciplinary Team Training*. Springer Publishing Company, New York.

Silver, G.A. (1958) Beyond general practice: the health team. *Yale Journal of Biology and Medicine*, 31, 29–38.

Spratley, J. (1990a) *Disease Prevention and Health Promotion in Primary Health*. Health Education Council, London.

Spratley, J. (1990b) *Joint Planning for the Development and Management of Disease Prevention and Health Promotion Strategies in Primary Health Care*. Health Education Council, London.

Storrie, J. (1992) Mastering interprofessionalism – an enquiry into the development of Masters programmes with an interprofessional focus. *Journal of Interprofessional Care*, 6(3), 253–60.

Szasz, G. (1969) Interprofessional education in the health sciences. *Milbank Memorial Fund Quarterly*, 47, 449–75.

Thomson, W. (1986) Multi-professional education for health professionals in the United Kingdom. In: *Multi-professional Education for Health Personnel in the European Region*. (eds J-F. d'Ivernois & V. Vodoratski). Annex 9. World Health Organization, Copenhagen.

Thwaites, M. (1993) Interprofessional education and training: a brief history. *CAIPE Bulletin*, No 6, pp. 2–3.

Tope, R. (1996) *Integrated Interdisciplinary Learning Between the Health and Social Care Professions: a Feasibility Study*. Avebury, Aldershot.

UNI Letter (1999) W.K. Kellogg Foundation. Temuco, Chile. Year 5. Number 16.

Vanclay, L. (1995) International developments. *CAIPE Bulletin*, No. 9. pp. 8–9.

Vinal, D. (1987) Interdisciplinary health care team care: nursing education in rural health settings. *Journal of Nursing Education*, 26(6), 258–9.

Wagner, C (1997) Germany explores scope for interprofessional education (a conference report). *Journal of Interprofessional Care*, 11(1), 110–11.

Walton, H.J. (1995) Multidisciplinary education. *Medical Education*, 29, 329–31.

World Federation for Medical Education (1988) The Edinburgh Declaration. *Lancet*, 332, (86008), 462.

World Federation for Medical Education (1994) Proceedings, World Summit on Medical Education, Edinburgh, 8–12 August 1993. *Medical Education*, 28 (Supplement 1).

World Health Organization (1973) *Continuing education for physicians*. Technical Report Series No. 534. World Health Organization, Geneva.

World Health Organization (1978) *The Alma Ata Declaration*. World Health Organization, Geneva.

World Health Organization (1987a) *Learning Together to Work Together for Health*. Technical Report No. 769. World Health Organization, Geneva.

World Health Organization (1987b) *Innovative Tracks at Established Institutions for the Education of Health Personnel: an Experimental Approach to Change Relevant to Health*. WHO Offset. Publication No. 101. World Health Organization, Geneva.

Further Reading

Barrows, H. & Tamblin, R. (1980) *Problem-Based Learning*. Springer Publications, New York.

Cherkasky, M. (1949) The Montefiore Hospital Home Care Program. *American Journal of Public Health*, **39**, 163–6.

Kovacic, L. (1988) Teamwork and multi-professional training programmes in health sector in Yugoslavia. In: *Multi-professional Education for Health Personnel in the European Region*. (eds J-F. d'Ivernois & V. Vodoratski). Annex 11. WHO, Copenhagen.

Lanara, V. (1988) Multi-professional training programmes and strategies for team training in Greece. In: *Multi-professional Education for Health Personnel in the European Region*. (eds J-F. d'Ivernois & V. Vodoratski). Annex 5. WHO, Copenhagen.

McMichael, P. & Gilloran, A. (1984a) *Exchanging Views: Courses in Collaboration*. Moray House College of Education, Edinburgh.

McMichael, P., Irvine, R. & Gilloran, A. (1984b) *Pathways to the Professions: Research Report*. Moray House College of Education, Edinburgh.

McMichael, P., Molleson, J. & Gilloran, A. (1984c) *Teaming up to Problem Solve*. Moray House College of Education, Edinburgh.

Magrab, P., Evans, P. & Hurrell, P. (1997) Integrated services for children and youth at risk: an international study of multidisciplinary training. *Journal of Interprofessional Care*, **11**(1), 99–108.

Makaram, S. (1995) Interprofessional cooperation. *Medical Education*, **29**, 65–9.

Rendas, A.B. (1988) Team training for health personnel in Portugal: an institutional point of view. In: *Multi-professional Education for Health Personnel in the European Region*. (eds J-F. d'Ivernois & V. Vodoratski). Annex 6. World Health Organization, Copenhagen.

Schmitt, M. (1994) USA: Focus on interprofessional practice, education and research. *Journal of Interprofessional Care*, **8**, 1.

Shigan, E. (1988) Combination of mono- and multidisciplinary courses in dynamic post-graduate training system of physicians in the USSR. In: *Multi-professional Education for Health Personnel in the European Region*. (eds J-F. d'Ivernois & V. Vodoratski). Annex 10. World Health Organization, Copenhagen.

World Health Organization (1976) Health manpower development Doc/A29/15. (unpublished). Presented to the 29th World Health Assembly. World Health Organization, Geneva.

Section IV
Postscript

In this section we sum up and suggest some next steps.

Andrea Wild and Geoffrey Meads

9 Summing Up

Next steps

It is time to close. There is little more to be said, but much more to be done. In some parts of the world like Latin America, as we have seen, cultural imperatives compel collaborative responses across previously neglected public services. In the UK, and other economically more developed countries, however, it is not so simple. Partnerships had been taken for granted prior to the advent of health systems modernising policies, on the presumption of individual, professional structures and status. These are now being rendered inadequate. The seeds of novel collaborations are being sown and it is vital in the new NHS, as elsewhere, that politicians do not pull up the young plants simply to see how they are progressing. Real roots are required here. The global perspectives point to a decade or more as the prerequisite for growth. Collaboration is the tortoise to the hare of competition.

We have argued that collaboration is a key element of the modernisation of health and social services, featuring heavily in policy across the globe and supported by a burgeoning development of interprofessional educational approaches. The outcome is potentially a much richer and lifelong learning experience for every professional. Whilst the benefits of collaboration are numerous, the dangers of non-collaboration can be grave. We have noted that collaboration enhances performance and contributes to the development of a more holistic model of health and social care, and discussed the new patterns of professional relationships emerging and the development of new professional profiles which reflect this collaborative imperative. Holistic care drives the integration of services – and organisations – and thence their professional constituents as well.

Final word

This book has been essentially about policy. Our hope, as this Blackwell's series moves on to look at interprofessional education in the next two volumes (Barr *et al.*, 2005, Freeth *et al.*, 2005), is that tomorrow's professionals will regard policy awareness and participation as key elements in collaborative learning and working throughout their careers. (Appendices A–C provide details of the three organisations waiting, ready and eager to respond to those whose collaboration appetites have been whetted).

Politics, people and their personalities, and principles with their sometimes surprisingly transient meanings, are the chief constituents of policy. An approach to each of these founded upon collaboration can make all the difference. Collaboration is a sound relationship in modernising health and social environments that also represents a global experiment in alternative patterns of professional relationships. We have sought to demonstrate the former and clarify the latter. The case for professional collaboration is neither simple nor straightforward, but it is relevant and, we would argue, it is right.

References

Barr, H., Koppel, I., Reeves, S., Freeth, D. & Hammick, M. (2005) *Effective Interprofessional Education: Evidence, Theory and Practice.* Blackwell, Oxford.

Freeth, D., Hammick, M., Barr, H. Koppel, I. & Reeves, S. (2005) *Effective Interprofessional Education: Development, Delivery and Evaluation.* Blackwell, Oxford.

Appendix 1: The UK Centre for the Advancement of Interprofessional Education (CAIPE)

CAIPE's purpose

CAIPE promotes and develops interprofessional education as a way to improve collaboration between practitioners and organisations in health and social care and as a means to improve integrated services to users.

CAIPE's work

An independent charity founded in 1987, CAIPE is a national resource. Its focus is on ways of enabling professions, in the university and workplace, to learn from and about each other, foster mutual respect, overcome barriers to collaboration and engender joint action. It promotes interprofessional learning which actively involves service users as essential partners. Closely associated with continuing work to establish the evidence base for interprofessional education, CAIPE is concerned to ensure the quality of this learning and to disseminate the best research.

CAIPE's relationship to members and other bodies

CAIPE's membership includes organisations and individuals in education, health and social care across the UK statutory, voluntary and independent sectors. Together they form a network for mutual support and stimulation. CAIPE maintains close links with an increasing number of like-minded organisations. Its relationship with the international *Journal of Interprofessional Care* is particularly important to members.

CAIPE offers:

- Information about interprofessional learning, including examples of good practice
- Opportunities to exchange experiences
- A lively programme of conferences and symposia
- Access to research
- Responses to policy documents on behalf of its members and representation nationally and internationally

CAIPE undertakes:

- Facilitation of work-based projects to improve collaboration and bring about change
- Partnership programmes with government, health and social care employers and educational providers
- Interprofessional Learning Workshops to prepare teachers, trainers, clinical supervisors and managers to work with interprofessional groups
- Mapping of interprofessional learning innovations in the UK and abroad

Recent and current work includes:

- Case studies in interprofessional learning for the Department of Health
- Facilitating new health and social care partnerships in London
- Interprofessional learning workshops for teachers, facilitators and clinical supervisors for a number of NHS primary care trusts, the acute sector and higher education
- A commission to work with a Teaching Primary Care Trust to generate a culture of interprofessional learning throughout its development

Services to members:

- Access to the CAIPE website
- A bulletin on recent developments in collaborative practice and education
- Response to enquiries for advice and information
- Access to research evidence about the content, methods and effectiveness of interprofessional learning

CAIPE
Kierran Cross
11 The Strand
London
WC2N 5HR
Tel: 020 7389 8014
Email: admin@caipe.org.uk
Website: www.caipe.org.uk

Appendix 2: The Relationships Foundation

The Relationships Foundation (established as a charity in 1993) believes that well-being, for individuals and society as a whole, is achieved through relationships. Strengthening relationships in public and private life is a central objective which it pursues in a variety of ways:

- Producing original research in key policy areas
- Implementing 'relational' ideas through high-level consultation and partner-ship with the private and public sector
- Pioneering fresh initiatives to tackle national policy problems
- Promoting quality of relationships as a priority in policy debate and working practice
- Helping individuals and organisations become more 'relational' through pub-lications, conferences, training and consultancy

Although still young, the Foundation has already established a successful track record in public life as a 'think and do tank'. It not only dares to think differently but also helps develop innovative approaches and solutions to key social and economic issues of the day: from unemployment and crime prevention to public services reform and peace-building.

The Relationships Foundation
Jubilee House
3 Hooper Street
Cambridge CB1 2NZ
Tel: 01223 566333
Fax: 01223 566359
Email: info@relationshipfoundation.org
Website: www.relationshipsfoundation.org

Appendix 3: International Primary Care Unit

Purpose

Applied research is the business of the Warwick University IPC Unit, with its principal targets for application being government health and social policies and modern local primary care organisations. The Unit seeks to ensure that the UK receives the transferable learning available from parallel contemporary developments in primary care policy and practice elsewhere. Above all, in using systematic criteria to identify which new concepts, models and processes can be converted into UK currencies, it looks to make real and rapid differences to public health and frontline services.

Approach

The Unit has adopted the principle of cross-sectoral alliances as its basic modus operandi. With participation and equity this was one of the World Health Organization's three founding principles for the modern primary health care movement in 1978. Collaboration between public, private and independent sector organisations is seen as an essential component of both the design and dissemination of all IPC Unit programmes. The Unit is a member of the WHO/WONCA supported global Network: Towards Unity for Health. Reflecting this tripartite relationship its principal partners include the Department of Health and local NHS primary care trusts, the Relationships Foundation and the NHSU. The Unit was established in April 2001 through initial grants from the PPP Trust, the West Midlands NHS Research Network and the UK Community Hospitals Association. It is a ten-year programme.

The Unit maintains a database for each of the 214 countries in the world, charting 'modernising' policy and organisational developments at state government level over the past five years. Sources for this database include the Department for International Development, the World Health Organization, the Department of Health's International Branch, the European Observatory and, of course, the relevant literature. After extensive discussions with UK corporate policy makers the following subject areas have been identified as the focus for transferable learning over the 2001–2005 period:

- models of local engagement
- combinations of health and social care
- relationships with corporate partners
- developments in interprofessional learning and collaboration
- alternative mixed funding initiatives

As policy issues, these five areas are characterised by a particular need for midterm progress in terms of ensuring effective organisational developments take place.

Using the framework of these subject areas and an interview structure derived from the critical questions posed by UK policy makers, up to three in depth case studies for each of the WHO's six regions are being undertaken by the Unit at any one time. The developmental learning from these is supplied directly to, for example, NHS primary care trusts, Department of Health modernisation teams and Workforce Directorates through masterclasses and local workshops. The present list of locations from which case study material is being obtained includes Chile, Peru, Greece, Georgia, Kyrgyzstan, the East African region and New Zealand. In almost every case major government led primary care reforms are closely associated with the politics of national regeneration. The Unit contributes regularly to relevant journals, NHS magazines and health care educational curricula design in conjunction with the UK Centre for the Advancement of Interprofessional Education.

Personnel
Dr Geoffrey Meads, Professor of Primary Care Organisational Research
Dr Frances Griffiths, NHS Career Scientist
Andrea Wild, Senior Research Fellow (IPC)
Michiyo Iwami, Research Fellow (IPC)
Dr Teresa Pawlikowska, Senior Clinical Lecturer (IPC)
Helen Tucker, Visiting Fellow (Community Health Care)
Catherine Beckett (Executive Assistant)
Plus Associates

International Primary Care Unit
Centre for Primary Health Care Studies, University of Warwick
CV4 7AL
Tel: +44 (0)24 7657 2950
Fax: +44 (0)24 7652 8375
Email: g.d.meads@warwick.ac.uk
andi.wild@warwick.ac.uk
m.iwami@warwick.ac.uk

Index

abuse, 63–4, 69–70
academic detailing, 51
Academy of Nurse Practitioners, 106
access, 87
accident and emergency, 87
accountability, 86, 90–94, 125
action research, 112–13
Addenbrookes Hospital, 89
Adelaide, University of, 138
adverse event (theoretical model), 63, 76
advocacy, 117, 123
Africa, 6, 38
agriculture, 143
Alazhari University, 108–09
Albania, 124
Algeria, 136, 143
Amadera Sintrez Hospital, 107
Arizona Charter, 38
Association for the Study of Medical
        Education, 139
Athens, 47
Audit Commission, 95, 115
autonomy, 29, 37, 40–42, 54
Australasia, 142–4
Australia, 8, 54, 112, 116, 127, 129, 136, 138,
        142–3
Austria, 38, 137

Bagnall, Pippa, x
balanced scorecard, 90
Barangay health worker, 50
Bamoko Initiative, 43, 131
Batchelder, Louise, x
Beckett, Catherine, x, 160
Belgium, 110, 137
Bird, Peter, x
Blair, Tony, 54
Bobigny, 140
Bolivia, 8, 44, 124
Brazil, 43, 110, 112, 116, 127, 132
Brent Social Services, 69
Bristol, Royal Infirmary, 63–7, 71–73,
        77
British Columbia, University of, 141
budgets, control of, 17–18, 92

California Medical School, 141
    State, 125
Cambridge, 86–9, 99–100, 158
Cameroons, 143
Canada, 8, 54, 124, 127, 136
cancer, 23, 87
Canning House, x
Care Trust, 109, 131–2
Carelift International, 12
care management, 9
Caribbean, 143
Carnegie Commission, 141
Centre for Advancement of
        Interprofessional Education, ix, 5–6,
        115, 139–44, 155–7, 160
children, 70, 87, 109
Chile, 28–9, 37, 42–3, 101, 160
choice, 101
Cishenau, 12
citizenship
    councils, 116
    panel, 87
Civil Society, 9, 11, 37, 96
Climbié, Victoria, 63, 67–82
clinical audit, 97
Coimbra, 10, 42, 107
collaboration, 15–35
Colorado, University of, 141
Colombia, 46–7, 143
Comités Locales de Administración de
        Salud (CLAS), 9, 53–4, 116
Commission
    for Healthcare Audit and Inspection
        (CHAI), 62
    for Health Improvement (CHI), 23, 86
    for Social Care Inspection (CSCI), 62,
        115
    for Public Patient Involvement, 116
commissioning, 31
commonality, 22
communication, styles of 20–21
community
    health, 31, 142
    oriented education, 108–09
    organisation, 8–9

Community-Based Education and Service (COBES), 12
community/campus partnerships, 142, 144
community development, 24–5, 143–4
complexity, 37, 40–42, 54
Concordis International, 6
Connexions, 30
continuity, 21
Consultant, 71–7
controls assurance, 41
coronary heart disease, 87
Costa Rica, 43–4, 130–31
crisis prevention, 61–82
Czechoslovakia, 137
Curtin, University of, 143

Dale, Jeremy, x
decentralisation, 8–9, 49, 54
deconcentration, 37, 53
Denmark, 48, 137
Deming, Edward, 93
Department for International Development (DFID), 37–8, 49, 159
Department of Health, 127, 159
development
   agenda, 105–06
   personal, 24
Diagnostic and Treatment Centre, 38, 47, 124, 128
directness, 20–21
distributional justice, 37, 43–5, 54
District Health System, 43
diversity, 55, 132
Dominican Republic, 143
drugs, 17, 88
duty, 9–10

Ealing, 68, 69, 70
Eastern Europe, 127
Eggers, Monica, x
Egypt, 136
Eldoret, 12
empowerment, 130
engineer, 143
enrichment, 37, 51–2, 54
equity, 37, 43–5, 54
Ethiopia, vii
European Network for the Development of Multi-Professional Education (EMPE), 137, 144
European Health Sciences, 140
European Union, 10, 12, 28, 47, 136–40
Everybody's Business, 38
Expert Patient, 110, 117

Fiji, 143
Finland, 37, 51–2, 110–11, 113, 137, 139–40
FONASA, 43
Foundation Hospital, 31, 131
France, 136–7, 140
Frisancho, Ariel, x
fundholding, 45
future generations, 54

Gateway Programme, 44
General Practice, 45, 52, 89, 98, 126
George Street, 131
Georgia
   State, 160
   Medical School, 141
Geriatric Interdisciplinary Team Training Program (GITT), 141
Germany, 8, 38, 52
Gezira University, 108–09
Ghana, 48
Ghent University, 110
Glaxo-Wellcome, 10
globalisation, 3–4, 37–9
Gorman, Paul, ix–x, xiv
Goteborg, University of, 140
governance, 8–9, 86, 95
   clinical, 3, 40–42, 97–8
   corporate, 40–41
Greenwich, University of, 12
Greece, 9, 37, 47–8, 127, 137, 160
Griffiths, Frances, ix, 160
Guinea, 51

Hallam, Sheffield, University of, 12
Haringey Social Services, 74–7, 81
Harrison, Victoria, x
Hartford Foundation, 141
Health Action Zone, 107–09
Health Education Authority, 137
Health Foundation, 6, 10
Health Maintenance Organisation, 45
Health Management Group, 124
Health Professions
   Council, 40
   Schools in Service to the Nation Program, 142
Helsinki, 52
Higgs Report, 93
Hong Kong, 131
Horder, John, ix, 139
Hungary, 137

Iceland, 140
independent assessment, 94
Indiana Medical School, 141

indicators, 86–92
Information Technology (IT), 88
integrated care, 3, 17, 37, 113–14
Inter-American Bank, 46
interdisciplinary annual conference, 142
intermediate care, 3, 9
Interprofessional Education (IPE), 105,
      108–15, 135–45
Israel, 9, 48, 129, 136
Italy, 105
Iwami, Michiyo, x, 160

Joint Evaluation Team, 5
Journal of Interprofessional Care, 155

Kaiser Permanente, 125
Karolinska Institute, 140
Kellogg Foundation, 46, 141–3
Kennedy Report, 61, 63–7, 71–82
Kenya, 12, 48, 109, 116
Kentucky Medical School, 141
Kings College, 12
Kings Fund, 89
Kuopio, University of, 140
Kyrygstan, 160

Laming, Lord, 67–80
Latin America, 143, 153
La Trobe, University of, 143
Learning and Teaching Support Network,
      139
Learning for Partnership Network, 139
learning organisation, 37, 48–50
learning together, 125–6, 135
Leech, Philip, viii
legislation
      Health Act, 107
      Health and Social Care Act, 107
Lewis, Mark, x
Limburg, 13
Linkoping, 138, 140
Lionis, Christos, x
Lisbon, 107
Lithuania, 12, 144
litigation, prevention of, 61–82
Local Strategic Partnership (LSP), 30, 88, 109
London, 131, 156
Londrina, University of, 112

Maastricht, 13, 49, 53, 112–13
managed care, 9, 37, 45, 51–2
managed competition, 45
management, 81, 93, 98–9
Manila, 50
market, 25

mediation, 5
Medicom, 4, 10
mental health, 63–4, 87, 105
Mexico, 44, 113, 130–31, 136
Michigan State Medical School, 141
Microsoft, 46
Middlesex Hospitals, 69–70, 75–7, 81
Minnesota, 141
modernisation, 7–13, 107–08, 160
Moldova, 12
Montreal, 131
multidisciplinary, colleges, 38
multiplexity, 21

Nairobi, vii, 10
Natal University, 112
National Association for Primary Care,
      10
   Institute for Clinical Excellence, 62, 117
   Service Framework, 111
      cancer, 23, 126
      Older People, 125–6
neighbourhood renewal, 108–09
Nepal, 136
Netherlands, 9, 45, 129
network, 17, 37, 46–8, 55, 130, 141–2
   for Community Partnerships for Health,
      49, 144, 159
Newcastle, 12, 112, 142
New Deal, 108
New Generations, 12
New Zealand
   Association for Medical Education, 143
   State, 160
Nevada Medical School, 141
New South Wales, University of, 142–3
NHS
   Alliance, 10, 116
   Direct, 129–30
   Plan, 36, 109, 116–17
   University, 112
Nicaragua, 130
Nokia, 51
non-accidental injury, 67–70
non-governmental organisation (NGO),
      10–12, 37, 53, 108
Nordic Network for Interprofessional
      Education (NIPNET), 140, 144
North America, 10, 131, 140–42
North Carolina Medical School, 141
Northumbria, University of, 12
Norway, 137, 139–40
Nuffield Foundation, 10
nurse practitioner, 142
Nyerere, Julius, vii

occupational therapy, 126–7
Office for Public Services Reform, 108
older people, 87
Opportunidades Sedesol, 130
Organisation for Economic Cooperation
      and Development (OECD) 136
organisational development, 24–5
Ortega Plaza, 50
Oulu Polytechnic, 140

paediatric cardiac surgery, 61, 64–7, 73–4, 77
Pakistan, 136
Pan-American Health Organisation, 46
Parity, 21–2
Paris-Nord University, 140
participation, 37, 40–42, 54, 110, 117
partners, 29–30, 95–6, 99–100
partnership
   duty of, 10, 54
   pentangle, 48–9
   for Quality Education, 142
patient
   centred, 32, 87, 102
   forums, 117
   Safety Agency, 62
   participation groups, 117
peer review, 97–9
Percy, David, x
performance, 3, 85–102
Performance and Innovation Unit (PIU), 30
performance management, 7, 41, 86–92
Periferiaka Systimata Ygias, 47
Peru, 8–9, 37, 53–4, 101, 116, 160
P.E.S.T., 91
Pew Charitable Trust Foundation, 141
Pfizer, 10
Philhealth, 49
Philippines, 8, 37, 49–50, 127, 136, 143
planning, 86–9, 91–2
police, 68, 69–71, 76–7, 79
policy, 30–31
Porto, 42
Portugal, 10, 37, 41–2, 107, 111, 128–9, 137
PPP Medical Trust, 6
pre-qualifying, 112
Presidential Inquiry, 64
prevention, 61–82
Primary Care Trust, 9, 31, 86–9, 107, 114,
      126, 130, 160
   Teaching PCT, 156
Primary Medical Services, 124
problem-based learning (PBL), 13, 112–13
professionalism, 27–8
public, 31–2
public health
   expenditure, 8

improvement, 3, 9–10, 23–4, 31
   stewardship, 8, 86
Public Service Agreement, 31

quality, 8, 37, 50–52, 55, 86
   Education Initiative, 142
   improvement, 6, 9–10, 23–4
   Institute of Health Care, 10, 107
Queensland, 143
Quezon City, 50

Rational Choice (theoretical model), 129
Rawlins, Sir Michael, 125
regulation, 8, 93, 97
Relational Health Care, 20–22
Relationships Foundation, vii–viii, 6, 15, 20
resource management, 8, 107
Richmond, Alan, x
risk
   assessment, 6
   management, 41, 101
Robert Wood Johnson Foundation, 142
Rockefeller Foundation, 141
Royal Colleges, 127
   of General Practitioners, 98, 106, 111
   of Nursing, 80, 116
   of Surgeons, 40
   of Psychiatrists, 29
   of Physicians, 40, 126
Russia, 137, 140
Rwanda, 5

sanitarian, 143
Santana, Paula, x
Santiago
   Catholic University, 43–5
   de Cali, 46
SARS, 39
Schluter, Michael, vii–viii
Scotland, 5
Scott, Michael Valdes, x
scrutiny, 101
seamless care, 17
Sector-Wide Approach, 37, 49–50, 55
Shanghai, 38
Sheffield Hallam University, 12
Sheffield, University of, 12
Shemasko System, 12
sickness fund, 45, 129
Singapore, 131
Singhealth, 125
Siripak, Chutatip, x
smoking cessation, 12, 30
Slovakia, 44
Social Exclusion Unit, 108
social inclusion, 23

social managerialism, 54
social services, 63, 67–79, 92
South Africa, 5, 39, 110, 112, 124, 143
South Australia Institute of Technology, 142
South Bank, University of, 12
Southampton, University of, 12
Spain, 38, 124, 137
Sri Lanka, 39
stakeholder, 4, 9, 90
STAKES, 52
strategy, 76–7, 90–91
  Unit, 30
substitution, 37, 43–6, 54
Sudan, 108–09, 136, 143
Supra Regional Service Advisory Group, 78
Sunderland, University of, 12
Sure Start, 30, 87
Sweden, 48, 52, 136–40
Swiss Cheese (theoretical model), 62, 75
Switzerland, 8, 37
Sydney, 137, 143
system, 30, 37
synthesis, 123, 132–3

Taiwan, 131
Tanzania, vii
targets, 89–93
taxonomy of collaboration, 27
teamwork, 17, 71–2, 111
Thailand, 39
Third Sector, 39
Thomas-Kilman, 26–7
Tountas, Mamas, x
transdiscipline, 46–8, 55
treasury, 31
Tromso University, 140
trust, 37, 53–5

TUFH, 38, 48–9, 116, 159
Turkey, 137

Uganda, 44, 127
UNESCO, 38
UNICEF, 38
United Bristol Hospital Trust, 63, 65
United States, 10, 38, 44, 106, 136, 143–4
unity, 132
unions, 28
USSR, 52, 137, 140
Utah Medical School, 141
Utrecht, 53

Vanersborg University, 140
Veterans Administration, 141
Virgin, 46

Warwick, University of, ix, 159–60
Western Cape University, 110
WONCA, 49, 159
workforce, 88
  Development Confederation, 4, 12
  practices, 12
World Bank, 10, 37–9, 111
  Development Report, 5
World Health Organisation, 37–8, 48, 55, 111, 113, 125, 135–6, 143–4, 159–60
World Federation of Medical Education (WFME), 136

Xerox, 95–6

Yatiri healer, 44
Yugoslavia, 137

Zambia, 48
Zimbabwe, 43
Zulu, 33

Printed in the United Kingdom
by Lightning Source UK Ltd.
133035UK00001BB/13/P